LOOK
GREAT
at
ANY AGE

OTHER BOOKS BY BRAD SCHOENFELD

Look Great Naked

Look Great Sleeveless

Sculpting Her Body Perfect

LOOK GREAT at ANY AGE

DEFY AGING, SLIM DOWN, AND OPTIMIZE HEALTH
IN JUST 60 MINUTES A WEEK

Brad Schoenfeld, CSCS

PRENTICE HALL PRESS
a member of Penguin Putnam Inc.
New York

Most Avery books are available at special quantity discounts for bulk purchase for sales promotions, premiums, fund-raising, and educational needs. Special books or book excerpts also can be created to fit special needs. For details, write Putnam Special Markets, 375 Hudson Street, New York, NY 10014.

a member of
Penguin Putnam Inc.
375 Hudson Street
New York, NY 10014
www.penguinputnam.com

Library of Congress Cataloging-in-Publication Data

Schoenfeld, Brad, date.
Look great at any age : defy aging, slim down, and optimize health
in just 60 minutes a week / Brad Schoenfeld.
p.   cm.
Includes index.
ISBN 0-7352-0331-8
1. Physical fitness for women.   2. Women—Health and hygiene.   I. Title.
GV482.S36   2003   2002030798
613.7'045—dc21

Printed in the United States of America
1   3   5   7   9   10   8   6   4   2

This book is printed on acid-free paper. ∞

BOOK DESIGN BY AMANDA DEWEY

Acknowledgments

To super-agent Bob Silverstein, for being a terrific agent as well as friend.

To Laura Shepherd, for bringing the project to life. It is a pleasure to work with an editor who is not only knowledgeable but also savvy.

To Christina Young, for your expert publicity efforts.

To Kristen Jennings, for your attention to detail and for keeping everything on schedule.

To my parents, for your continual support.

To all my clients at the Personal Training Center for Women, past and present, for helping me perfect the High-Energy Fitness system and furthering my quest for self-actualization.

To all the trainers who have worked at the Personal Training Center for Women, past and present, for helping me make a positive impact on the lives of so many.

To Barbara Kaufman, Vilma Lusardi, and Annette Saleski. You're not only great models, but also true fitness inspirations.

To Joe Weider, for helping to bring fitness into the mainstream and expanding my knowledge in the early years.

To all the professors of nutrition and exercise science who, through your teachings and writings, have furthered my knowledge in a complex field.

Contents

Introduction

The voice on the other end of the phone asked a question that seemed rather strange at the time: "Do you work with *older* women?"

"Of course," I replied, still not fully comprehending the nature of her question. "I've been a personal trainer for many years and have helped women as old as eighty realize their fitness goals."

There was a slight pause, then the woman went on to relate her history: Her name was Susan, and she had just celebrated her fifty-second birthday. Susan had never exercised a day in her life, conceding that her most strenuous chore was lifting the grocery packages from the shopping cart into her car! She was now thirty pounds over her ideal weight, had difficulty picking up her grandson, and was constantly feeling fatigued. Moreover, she was now going through menopause, which was creating a great deal of stress in her life as well as bringing her inevitable mortality into the forefront of her mind.

Despite understanding that she had to do *something* to counteract her predicament, Susan was very wary about commencing an exercise program. She questioned whether she was even a viable candidate to perform physical activity, asking, "Do you think it's too late for me to start working out?" The concept of fitness was totally foreign to her, and she was quite fearful of the prospect of working out.

Unfortunately, there is still a prevailing reluctance on the part of many women, especially those over forty, to lift weights. Some have a subconscious, deep-rooted fear of exercise that has been ingrained since childhood. Others still cling to the misconception that strength training is reserved for buffed hardbodies with bulging biceps and six-pack abs. Whatever their reasons, these women are missing out on the most important activity they can perform.

Plain and simply, strength training is the fountain of youth, a tried-and-true remedy that really can reverse the aging process. Without question, no other activity has more of an impact on your overall health and well-being. Sure, aerobic exercise is important—it conditions the cardiovascular system and helps to expedite fat loss. However, all things considered, nothing compares to the myriad benefits that are derived from a dedicated strength-training program including improved strength, increased bone density, better posture, elevated metabolism, reduced stress, and, of course, a firm, toned body that looks great—both in and out of clothing.

This book provides a tried-and-true fitness solution for looking and feeling your very best. It's a cutting-edge program that's designed to provide maximum results in a minimal amount of time. The routine is home based; with just a set of dumbbells and a bench, you're ready to work out.

Best of all, the program is very time efficient. The entire routine should take you about twenty minutes to perform. As you'll see, it's the *quality*, not the *quantity*, of training that builds a terrific physique. In the case of exercise, less really is more. Considering the minimal time commitment involved, you can't use the excuse that it's impossible to fit a workout into your busy schedule.

The book is divided into three parts:

Part I explores the major issues that have an impact on health and appearance. Specific chapters are devoted to the effects of exercise on body fat, bone density, cardiovascular function, and mental health. Each chapter is punctuated with interesting anecdotes from personal experiences with clients at my private women's training facility (yes, they are all true!).

Part II details the Look Great at Any Age exercise regimen. I provide a pre-exercise checklist that goes over everything you need to know before you start training, a comprehensive explanation of the training protocols associated with the program, and three different sample workout routines.

Part III outlines the Look Great at Any Age nutritional program. Proper nutrition is vital to achieving a healthy body—at least as important as exercise. I discuss the realities of protein, carbs, and fats, providing strategies for developing a practical eating plan. Many dietary inaccuracies and myths are debunked. There are no gimmicks here: only scientifically based concepts that have been proven to work. A seven-day sample diet is included to get you on the right track.

In sum, everything you need to get on the road to a new you is here in this book. If you put in the effort, results are guaranteed.

Finally, in case you were wondering . . . Susan became my client and embraced a fitness lifestyle. She started exercising on a regular basis and drastically changed her nutritional habits. In the six months that I've worked with her, she is down to her ideal body weight, is stronger than her husband, is in perfect medical health, and, best of all, looks and feels better than she has in twenty years!

THE
AGING
CONCERN

PART ONE

CHAPTER 1

The Skinny on Fat

Americans are forever trying to win the battle of the bulge; unfortunately, we seem to be losing the war. Despite spending billions a year on weight-loss aids, more than two-thirds of the country's population is overweight. Even more alarming, approximately 20 percent of the population is considered clinically obese. By all accounts, the situation has reached epidemic proportions.

To most people, fat is a mysterious entity that brings about more questions than answers. What causes fat storage? How is fat burned? Why are some areas more resistant to fat loss than others? To unlock these mysteries, a little physiology lesson is in order.

Fat is contained in cells called *adipocytes*. Adipocytes are pliable storehouses that either shrink or expand to accommodate fatty deposits. They are present in virtually every part of the body. There is a direct correlation between the size of adipocytes and obesity: the larger your adipocytes, the fatter you appear. However, although adipocytes can be reduced in size, they can't be completely eliminated. The reality is, once adipocytes form, you are stuck with them for life.

On the surface of each adipocyte are tiny *receptors* that control the storage and release of fat from the cell. Receptors can be likened to doorways; they either allow fat into or out of adipocytes. There are two basic types of fat receptors: alpha-2 receptors and beta receptors. Taking the doorway analogy a step further, alpha-2 receptors are the "entrances" that let fat into adipocytes for long-term storage while beta receptors are the "exits" that let fat out of adipocytes to be burned for energy. Depending on various physiologic factors (hormonal stimulus, enzymatic activity, caloric availability, etc.), these receptors ultimately determine whether body fat is gained or lost.

Because of the distribution of receptors, women have an especially difficult time staying lean. It has been shown that specific adipocytes—especially the ones in a woman's lower body—have a higher percentage of alpha receptors to beta receptors (as high as six to one, by some estimates) and therefore tend to hoard fat and hold on to it. Hence, women are the fatter sex; on average, they carry about double the amount of fat as their male counterparts.

The accumulation of body fat generally begins at the onset of puberty. During this period, there is a surge in the production of estrogen. Estrogen is a hormone that promotes secondary female sex characteristics. Among its many functions, estrogen is integrally involved in the storage of body fat. Specifically, it exerts a regional influence on lipoprotein lipase—an enzyme that signals the body to store fat. In lower body adipocytes, estrogen stimulates lipoprotein lipase activity, causing fat to accumulate in this area. Conversely, estrogen has the opposite effect in the upper body, where it actually suppresses the activity of lipoprotein lipase and thereby impedes fat deposition. This site-specific response diverts fat away from the torso and into the lower body, producing the rounded features normally associated with a feminine physique.

FAT AND PREGNANCY

When a woman becomes pregnant, body fat levels rise even farther. Fat is a primary energy source used for fetal development. It helps to nourish the fetus and fuel the growth and maturation of fetal organs, vessels, and bones. In order to support these extra energy requirements, the body attempts to mobilize as much fat as possible. It does so by secreting a large amount of progesterone—a hormone that increases appetite. Progesterone levels remain elevated throughout pregnancy, inducing the intense cravings commonly associated with childbirth.

In addition, there is a rapid proliferation of adipocytes. Millions of new fat cells are created, with most of them deposited in the lower-body region. All told, the average weight gain associated with pregnancy approaches thirty pounds—much of it in the form of fat. And these effects are exacerbated with multiple pregnancies; after the second or third child, losing postpartum weight becomes more and more problematic.

Compounding matters is the fact that women are now having children later in life. Advances in medical technology have made it possible to conceive through artificial insemination, allowing millions of aging baby boomers to experience the joys of childbirth. It now is not unusual for a woman to become pregnant in her mid-forties—an occurrence virtually unheard-of just a few decades ago.

But women who conceive in midlife often face a greater challenge to get back into shape after delivery. They find that the body just doesn't snap back as easily as it once did and accumulated body fat seems to be especially hard to get rid of.

FAT AND AGING

The aging process also has a negative effect on body composition. This is reflected in the so-called 20/20, 30/30, rule: statistics show that the typical woman has approximately 20 percent body fat at the age of twenty, 30 percent at the age of thirty, and so on. Thus, unless she does something to combat the process, by the time a woman reaches her fiftieth birthday, roughly half of her body will be composed of fat.

The age-related accretion of body fat is largely due to a loss of muscle tissue. You see, women lose roughly 1 percent of their muscle mass each year after the age of thirty and continue to do so throughout the rest of their lives. Muscle is the most metabolically active tissue in the body; the more you have, the more calories you burn. That's why a reduction of muscle progressively slows metabolism, causing a gradual but steady increase in body fat.

In addition, changes that take place in the body during menopause cause a shift in the distribution of body fat. Because of a decline in estrogen levels, fat begins to accumulate to a greater degree in the midsection. The hourglass figure is replaced by the male "android" shape, and increased abdominal fat is the upshot.

CELLULITE

Body fat is directly associated with another unwanted malady: cellulite. In common terms, cellulite is the "orange peel" look that appears on the surface of skin. Although these pockets of fat can form anywhere on the body, they most often manifest themselves in the butt and thighs. The triceps (backs of the upper arms) and the abdominal region also are susceptible, albeit to a lesser degree.

Despite the claims of various hucksters, cellulite is a genetic condition that can't be purged by magic creams or potions. You see, cellulite tends to be hereditary; if your mother and siblings are afflicted, the chances are good that you will be too. As is true of your height, eye color, and hair texture, genetics dictate where fat is deposited and the semblance that it takes on your body. Hence, while some women can be obese with little evidence of cellulite, others can be relatively thin and have cottage-cheese thighs. This is simply the luck of the draw. If you picked good parents, you might escape the big C. If not . . .

Interestingly, men rarely develop cellulite. This is due to the composition of human skin. The skin and its underlying tissue have three fundamental layers: The top layer is composed of a cellular-based tissue called the dermis. Its primary purpose is to protect your body from outside contaminants. The middle layer is made up of fibrous connective tissue called superficial fascia. It is substantially thicker than the dermis and acts like an internal stocking to support the skin. The lower layer is made up of adipose tissue—plain old fat. It has several functions including insulating the body, padding the internal organs, and providing a source of long-term energy.

You're probably wondering how this information applies to cellulite. Well, the superficial fascia is responsible for holding body fat in place. In men, the superficial fascia is arranged in a crisscross pattern that is strong and consistent. Accordingly, fat is contained in a uniform manner below the skin, leaving the skin surface smooth and supple. In women, however, the superficial fascia tends to be irregular and discontinuous. It has a vertical distribution, forming honeycomb-like patterns beneath the dermis. Hence, when fat accumulates, it pushes up toward the skin's surface in clusters, giving the skin the lumpy, dimpled appearance commonly known as cellulite.

Cellulite is further exacerbated by the localized accumulation of lymphatic fluid. Research has shown that cellulite contains an abundance of glycosaminoglycans—a carbohydrate-based compound that has high water-attracting properties. Glycosaminoglycans draw fluid into fatty tissue, causing extensive swelling in cellulite-affected areas. This heightens the density of cellulite, making it heavy and voluminous.

Given that cellulite is related to the structural composition of connective tissue, it's easy to see why it's impossible for a cream to eradicate the problem; there simply is no way that an externally applied solution can penetrate the skin and "reconfigure" the underlying connective tissue.

FAT AND HEALTH

While the detrimental effects of excessive body fat on external appearance are readily apparent, the internal effects sometimes go overlooked. But make no mistake, a high degree of body fat has implications beyond aesthetics—it also has a serious impact on overall health. Obese people have about twice the chronic health problems of those of normal weight. Perhaps more alarmingly, the health risks of obesity are even greater than those of smokers and heavy drinkers!

The statistics are ominous. Studies show that women who gain ten to forty pounds in midlife have a substantially increased risk of suffering heart attacks. With each increment of weight gain, coronary risk rises exponentially: Those who gain eleven to eighteen pounds have a 25 percent greater risk; those who gain eighteen to twenty five pounds have a 60 percent greater risk; and those who gain more than 25 pounds have up to a 300 percent greater risk.

Obesity also has been linked to many types of cancer. Although the exact causes are not fully understood, the relationship between excess body fat and cancer is indisputable. Specifically, studies have shown that those who are overweight have an increased risk of cancer of the endometrium, breast, kidneys, colon, and pancreas.

In addition, obesity can cause serious musculoskeletal problems. Having excess body fat is like carrying around a suitcase all day. It places tremendous demands on the musculoskeletal system, transferring undue stress to joints and connective tissue. Estimates show that each one-pound increase in body weight causes a three-pound increase in stress to joints. This can directly lead to lower-back pain, osteoarthritis, and other joint-related anomalies.

THE DIET PARADOX

Most people try to lose weight through diet alone, sometimes starving themselves to shed the extra pounds. What a mistake! In the absence of exercise, dieting breaks down crucial muscle tissue. Sure, cutting calories causes you to lose fat, but it results in the loss of a significant amount of muscle, too. During times of caloric restriction, as when dieting, the body begins to rely on its endogenous (internal) amino acid pool for energy. Amino acids are derived from protein, and the body's main source of endogenous protein is muscle tissue. Studies have shown that up to 45 percent of the energy deficit from a calorie-restricted diet is caused by the burning of muscle for fuel—a fact that can account for as much as one pound a week of muscle loss.

What makes matters worse is that dieting causes the thyroid gland to become sluggish, resulting in an even further decrease in metabolic rate and reducing the body's ability to burn calories. This creates a vicious cycle where calorie consumption must be continually decreased in order to sustain

I've been fat all my life," Julie uttered tearfully, trying her best to contain her emotions. "I've been through every diet imaginable, and nothing has ever worked. A few times I was able to lose about thirty pounds, but I always gained it back shortly thereafter . . ."

At five foot seven, Julie weighed at least three hundred pounds (she would not let me weigh her because she had broken a scale in another facility causing great embarrassment). She was fifty-one years old, and the effects of carrying all this extra weight over the years were beginning to take a toll on her health.

Julie became one of my first clients after the opening of my center. She was a hard worker who desperately wanted to get her condition under control. Combined with a sensible nutritional plan, I put Julie on the Look Great at Any Age program. Due to her weight, she was severely limited when we began. However, she did not let this get in the way of attaining her ultimate goal.

Over time, Julie's weight loss was steady, if not spectacular. Each month, her body showed visible change. After two years, Julie had gotten her weight down to 150 pounds—she was ecstatic! Better still, she has been able to keep the weight off ever since: an accomplishment that escapes the great majority of dieters.

weight loss. After a while, your diet will hit a plateau, and the body simply becomes resistant to any more weight loss. Inevitably, when the diet is discontinued, body weight balloons back up—often in excess of the original starting point. This is why women who yo-yo diet (try every new diet that comes into vogue) seem to have such difficulty achieving lasting weight loss.

THE LOOK GREAT AT ANY AGE PRESCRIPTION

The only realistic way to lose body fat is to combine diet with exercise (especially weight training). Unfortunately, many overweight women shy away from strength training, clinging to the belief that you shouldn't lift weights until you get down to your ideal body weight. I hear the same statement over and over again: "Lifting weights will only end up making me look fatter and bulkier. So I'm going to diet down first, then I'll tone up." This is simply bad reasoning! In order to lose body fat and, more important, keep it off permanently, you need to build muscle. Muscle increases your metabolic rate, which directly aids in burning fat for fuel. For each pound of muscle added to your body, you burn up to an additional 50 calories a day. Better yet, you're burning these calories on a continual basis, even when you're lying on the couch watching your favorite TV program! To put this in perspective, by gaining a mere five pounds of lean muscle (which, if you're a beginner, can be accomplished in a matter of months), you'll burn an additional 1,750 calories a week. Assuming you keep food consumption constant, those five pounds of muscle will result in a net loss of about twenty-five pounds in just one year's time!

So, to lose body fat, weight training isn't an option—it's a necessity. Performing aerobic activities is fine for helping to burn calories, but it does virtually nothing to increase muscle. Therefore, the effect on resting metabolism is negligible. Aerobic exercise increases caloric expenditure only during the performance of the activity itself (and for a short time postworkout).

Thus, while aerobics are a good adjunct to lifting weights, they are not a viable substitute. As a testament to this fact, consider that many bodybuilders never do any form of aerobic exercise, yet they remain extremely lean year-round. Their extensive muscularity provides such a great metabolic effect that aerobics simply aren't necessary. Now this isn't to say that you need to develop "large" muscles, just that it's beneficial to maintain a healthy amount of lean tissue.

Also, no exercise can localize fat loss. While weight training can target and tone certain muscles, there simply is no way to "spot-reduce" body fat; it's a physiologic impossibility. Despite the inflated claims made by certain unscrupulous hucksters, individual exercises can't slim down a specific area of your body—no matter how often or intensely you perform the movement. All the sit-ups in the world won't give you a flat stomach; no amount of lower-body exercises will directly diminish the size of your thighs. In reality, trying to eradicate your problem areas with targeted movements is literally an exercise in futility.

In order to appreciate why spot reduction doesn't work, it is necessary to understand the fat-burning process. When you exercise, fat stores are mobilized and are then transported via the blood to be used in target tissues for energy. Because fatty acids must travel through the circulatory system—a time-consuming event—it is just as efficient for your body to utilize fat from one area as it is another. In other words, the proximity of fat cells to the working muscles is completely irrelevant from an energy standpoint. Since the body can't preferentially use fat from a particular area, it simply draws from adipocytes in all regions of the body including the face, trunk, and extremities. The bottom line: Perform the routine as described and you'll ultimately lose unwanted body fat, even from those hard-to-lose areas. And by adding lean muscle to cellulite-ridden body parts, you'll help to smooth out the region and provide a supporting structure that gives it a firm, toned appearance. While this won't necessarily eradicate cellulite, it certainly will diminish its manifestation.

Following the Look Great at Any Age program is the surest way to lose body fat and achieve lasting weight management. In addition to promoting muscle-induced increases to resting metabolic rate, it also brings about a phenomenon called excess postexercise oxygen consumption (EPOC). Simply stated, EPOC means that calories are burned at an accelerated rate following a workout session. This is over and above your resting metabolism.

EPOC is the body's way of restoring equilibrium. The primary mechanism here is oxygen. During exercise, large amounts of oxygen are used to fuel performance. This creates an "oxygen debt" that needs to be "repaid" after the completion of training. Because oxygen is directly involved in fat burning, EPOC can bring about tangible improvements in body composition. In fact, EPOC results in an increase of caloric expenditure by more than 13 percent after intense exercise with an elevation in metabolism seen for more than sixteen hours, postworkout!

CHAPTER 2

Have Some Heart

Of all the muscles in your body, none is more important than your heart. That's right, the heart is a muscle—a fact that many people seem to forget. But the heart has certain characteristics that set it apart from the skeletal muscles. Namely, unlike the biceps or pectorals, the heart can't simply take a rest when it's tired. It must work continually throughout the day, beating in a controlled, rhythmic fashion. This process is regulated by internal *pacemakers,* which send electrical impulses to various cardiac *nodes.* Provided that there are no electrical disturbances, a consistent heart rate is maintained depending on activity levels (usually at a pace of around 60 to 80 beats per minute under resting conditions).

From a practical standpoint, the heart is basically a glorified pump. It interfaces with arteries and veins to transport blood throughout the body. Arteries branch out into tiny vessels called *capillaries,* which deliver oxygen-rich blood to the muscles and internal organs. After these tissues extract the oxygen, deoxygenated blood is then returned to the heart through the veins, forming the closed-loop network known as the cardiovascular system.

In many ways, the function of the cardiovascular system can be compared to that of a hot tub. A hot tub is comprised of a pump (your heart), some pipes (your arteries), and water (your blood). The pump drives water through the pipes and into the tub. The water is then recirculated, traveling back through the pipes, where it again enters the pump. The process repeats again and again, allowing a steady flow of filtered water through the tub's jets.

CARDIOVASCULAR DISEASE

As you undoubtedly know, the cardiovascular system is susceptible to a multitude of diseases. Fortunately, women are somewhat protected from cardiovascular illness during the premenopausal years. This is largely due to the cardioprotective effects of estrogen. But the bad news is that after the onset of menopause, this protection disappears, leaving women extremely vulnerable to cardiovascular problems. In fact, heart attacks are now the leading cause of death in women, accounting for about one-third of all fatalities. Moreover, since 1984, the number of female-related cardiovascular fatalities has actually exceeded that of men. This belies the prevailing misconception that coronary artery disease is predominantly a male-oriented affliction.

Although many factors contribute to the onset of cardiovascular disease, three are of particular concern with respect to fitness: insulin resistance, hypertension, and high cholesterol. Let's discuss each of these risk factors in detail.

INSULIN RESISTANCE

Your body's ability to regulate blood sugar (called glucose tolerance) is a major risk factor in the onset of cardiovascular disease. Blood sugar is derived from the food that you eat. After a meal, your body breaks down carbohydrates (and, to a lesser extent, protein and fats) into glucose, a simple sugar, so that it can be used for fuel. The glucose then circulates throughout the bloodstream until it is taken up in the cells.

Insulin, a pancreatic hormone, is the primary regulator of blood sugar. When blood-sugar levels rise, the beta cells of the pancreas secrete insulin to drive glucose into cells. The main targets of insulin are muscle and adipose tissue (fat cells). These tissues contain transporter proteins called GLUT4, which interact with insulin to facilitate glucose uptake. Think of GLUT4 like glucose ferries; they rise to the cell surface to meet sugar molecules and then shuttle them to the inside of the cell.

Under certain circumstances, however, cells lose some of their capacity to take in glucose. This condition, called insulin resistance, is thought to be the cause of "Syndrome X"—a group of metabolic afflictions (including increased cholesterol, elevated blood pressure, and increased abdominal fat deposits) that have been implicated in a host of cardiovascular anomalies.

Over time, incessant insulin resistance leads to diabetes—a potentially lethal disease that affects more than sixteen million Americans. In addition to contributing to heart attacks and strokes (diabetics are four times as likely to suffer a cardiovascular event), diabetes also brings about a variety of other complications including blindness, kidney failure, and nerve damage. It can even lead to gangrene, particularly of the legs and feet, often resulting in amputation of the lower extremities.

For reasons that aren't completely clear, diabetes is more lethal in women than it is in men. Diabetic women have a sevenfold increase in cardiovascular risk, as compared to only a threefold increase in men. Given that approximately 60 percent of all reported cases occur in women, these statistics are particularly ominous.

There are two basic classifications of diabetes. The first, Type 1 diabetes (a.k.a. insulin-dependent diabetes mellitis), is a congenital disease; it occurs during childhood or adolescence and persists throughout life. In Type 1 diabetes, the body destroys its own pancreatic beta cells so that insulin cannot be produced. Since there is no cure as yet, those afflicted must take daily insulin injections for survival.

The other kind of diabetes is called Type 2 diabetes (a.k.a. non-insulin-dependent diabetes). As opposed to Type 1 diabetes, it is an acquired disease that can become manifest at any age. Comprising 90 percent of all cases, it is far and away the most common form of diabetes. Here, the beta cells of the pancreas can produce insulin but the insulin is not able to effectively clear blood sugar from circulation.

Contrary to popular belief, the primary cause of Type 2 diabetes isn't a result of the inability of insulin to bind to target cells. Rather, it is caused by a breakdown in GLUT4 function. In effect, there is a "shortcircuit" in the insulin signal that normally causes GLUT4 to rise to the cell surface. Without the assistance of GLUT4, glucose simply cannot enter the cells. Consequently, sugar just keeps circulating in the bloodstream, leading to the devastating complications associated with diabetes.

HYPERTENSION

High blood pressure—an increase in the force of blood against the walls of your arteries—is another significant risk factor in cardiovascular disease. Blood pressure is measured by placing a cuff on the upper arm and taking a reading on a special mercury-containing device. A reading has two numerical components and is expressed as a ratio in millimeters of mercury (mm/Hg): The first number is the *systolic* pressure, which measures the pressure against your arteries when your heart contracts; the second number represents the *diastolic* pressure, which measures the pressure against your arteries when your heart is at rest.

The body has an internal feedback mechanism that constantly regulates blood pressure. It uses specialized sensors (called baroreceptors) to accomplish this task. The baroreceptors are located primarily in the carotid arteries of the neck, which interconnect with the heart and blood vessels through a series of nerves. They operate much like a thermostat: If blood pressure falls too low, the sensors send neural impulses to increase heart rate and thereby ensure adequate flow to bodily tissues; if blood pressure rises significantly, the sensors signal the heart to reduce cardiac output so that vessels aren't unduly stressed.

When the system is operating properly, the baroreceptors allow blood pressure to rise and fall within a range that best accommodates the immediate demands on the body. But sometimes the baroreceptors malfunction and lose their ability to maintain normal blood pressure. In effect, the "thermostat" gets reset at a higher level causing blood pressure to remain consistently elevated, a condition known as hypertension. Clinically speaking, hypertension is defined as a resting blood pressure where the systolic component is greater than 140 and/or the diastolic component is greater than 90 (i.e., 140/90 mm/Hg).

To appreciate how hypertension affects the cardiovascular system, let's revisit the hot-tub analogy. In a hot tub, water is constantly flowing through the pipes at a given pressure. Provided that the water pressure is regulated, everything runs smoothly. But if the water pressure remains significantly increased for a prolonged period of time, the pipes become unduly stressed. The end result is that either the pipes (your arteries) burst or the pump (your heart) gives out, causing a complete breakdown of the hot tub (your body).

Realize, though, that your blood pressure is constantly rising and falling throughout the day depending on various lifestyle factors. Many incidents (including intense exercise) can cause a transient rise in blood pressure, but these spikes generally pose little threat to your health. On the other hand, chronic hypertension can have dire consequences. It is both a sign, as well as a causal factor, in heart attacks, strokes, and congestive heart failure. Given that nearly 50 million Americans are classified as hypertensive, it's no wonder that high blood pressure is the leading associated cause of death and disability in Westernized societies.

CHOLESTEROL

High cholesterol is perhaps the biggest risk factor for cardiovascular disease. The mere mention of the words conjures up images of clogged arteries. But cholesterol isn't necessarily the detriment that it's often perceived to be. In fact, it is an essential component in many biological functions. It is an integral constituent in cell membranes, acts as a precursor to many hormones (including the sex hormones estrogen and testosterone, amongst others), and forms the basis of bile salts that aid in the digestion and absorption of fat and fat-soluble vitamins in the intestine.

The cholesterol in your body is derived from dietary sources as well as from internal production. But contrary to popular belief, consuming cholesterol-laden foods generally has little effect on your cholesterol profile (except for a small percentage of people who are predisposed to very high cholesterol levels). This is due to the body's ability to increase and decrease its own internal cholesterol production based on the amount of cholesterol consumed in the diet—a so-called *negative feedback loop*.

From a physiologic perspective, cholesterol is a waxy, fatlike substance. Because of its fatty composition, cholesterol can't directly mix with water. Hence, it must be packaged into protein-based compounds called lipoproteins for transport through the bloodstream, where it is taken up for use in various target tissues.

While there are several different classifications of lipoproteins, the most notable are the low-density lipoproteins (LDL) and high-density lipoproteins (HDL). LDL is the "bad cholesterol" commonly associated with heart disease. When excessive amounts of LDL circulate in the bloodstream, they attach themselves to the lining of the arteries. Over time, these cholesterol deposits become oxidized (think of rust on the inside of a pipe), causing localized inflammation. The body responds to the inflammation by secreting white blood cells, known as macrophages, to initiate healing. But instead of helping the situation, the macrophages ultimately become trapped in the inflamed area and develop into *foam cells,* which cause the formation of a plaque. This sets off a chain reaction where the body keeps sending more and more macrophages to the area, adding to the size of the plaque. Eventually, the plaque mass clogs up the artery, impeding blood flow. In severe cases, the artery can become completely blocked, cutting off all circulation to the heart, brain, legs, or other organs.

HDL, on the other hand, is considered the "good cholesterol." It acts as a cholesterol scavenger, carrying surplus cholesterol from the tissues back to the liver. Cholesterol is then either excreted in the feces or converted into bile acids, which are important compounds that act as emulsifying agents in the gut in the digestion of fats and oils. Accordingly, plasma HDL concentrations are inversely related to coronary artery disease—the greater the amount of HDL, the lower the incidence of heart attacks and vice versa.

Studies have repeatedly shown that a high amount of blood cholesterol (a.k.a. hypercholesterolemia) is detrimental to cardiovascular health. The current advice is to maintain a blood cholesterol level below 200—any more and you increase your risk of cardiovascular illness. Alarmingly, more than half of all women over the age of fifty-five have a total cholesterol level that exceeds 240 mg/dl.

While having a low total cholesterol level is certainly important, a potentially more meaningful indicator of cardiac risk is the ratio of total cholesterol to HDL. This ratio takes into account the cardioprotective benefits of HDL—a factor that's completely ignored in a basic cholesterol profile. Ideally, your cholesterol/HDL ratio should be 4 or less, which would indicate that your body is efficiently disposing of harmful LDLs.

THE LOOK GREAT AT ANY AGE PRESCRIPTION

The Look Great at Any Age program is designed to be a heart-healthy regimen. By performing the routine on a regular basis, you'll go a long way toward staving off the ravages of cardiovascular disease. In fact, with dedication and effort, you can even reverse some of the damage done to your peripheral vascular system as a result of a sedentary lifestyle.

First and foremost, the program helps to make your heart stronger. In the same way that exercise causes your biceps to develop, regimented training strengthens your heart so it's better able to sustain high-force pressures. As your heart muscle gets stronger and thicker, it can better withstand the demands of strenuous activities. Given that heart attacks are often associated with overexertion (such as shoveling snow, moving a heavy object, etc.), the implications are clear: A stronger heart that can endure these activities is a healthier heart.

In addition, the fast-paced nature of the program produces an aerobic effect that improves coronary circulation. Not only do your major coronary vessels increase in size, but so do your collateral arteries, which supply an alternative means of blood flow to the heart if there is a coronary blockage. Further, your network of capillaries—tiny blood vessels that surround and nourish the heart—expand in both size and number. On the whole, blood flow is greater to all regions of the heart, providing better oxygen and nutrient delivery to cellular tissues.

Other cardiovascular benefits of the program are achieved indirectly. For one, the program helps to improve glucose tolerance. These improvements are accomplished, in part, by increasing the sensitivity of GLUT4—the transporters responsible for bringing glucose into cells. You see, glucose is the primary source of muscular energy for high-energy activities. As you train, muscular contractions "wake up" GLUT4, allowing your muscles to take in glucose at an accelerated rate—up to five times more than under resting conditions—to fuel activity.

Better yet, your body is able to use glucose for up to forty-eight hours after a workout. Because glucose is depleted during training, your muscles are literally starved for carbohydrate in the postexercise period. Enzymes are produced to fill the need quickly, and glucose is shuttled into muscles in such an expedient fashion that insulin is not needed in great amounts. The bottom line is that blood-sugar levels are stabilized, decreasing the risk of developing Type 2 diabetes by as much as 40 percent.

Another heart-healthy aspect of the Look Great at Any Age program is its effect on lowering and preventing the incidence of hypertension. After exercise, blood pressure is temporarily reduced to below resting levels—a phenomenon referred to as the *hypotensive response*. This is thought to be related to the pooling of blood in the extremities, which reduces overall blood volume and thereby causes a decline in blood pressure. Although the most significant reductions are noted in the first few hours after a session, the lingering effects can last as long as twenty-four hours.

Over time, exercise has a profound impact on resting blood pressure. Physically fit people have a 35 percent reduced incidence of hypertension. In those who exercise and have mild to moderate hypertension, blood pressure is substantially lowered—enough, in many cases, to reduce significantly the required dosage of, if not completely eliminate the need for, drug therapy. Exercise is medicine!

Last but not least, the Look Great at Any Age program appreciably improves blood cholesterol. Regular exercise brings about a reduction in total cholesterol levels, a decline in LDL (the "bad" cholesterol) levels, an increase in HDL (the good "cholesterol") levels, and, most important, a decrease in the total cholesterol/HDL ratio.

Because the program is rigorous, the effects on HDL levels are particularly dramatic. Studies show that high-intensity training regimens have the greatest impact on increasing HDL levels. Since HDL is responsible for clearing particles that cause many plaques from the bloodstream, there is a diminished potential for hardening of the arteries.

A final word: For those who already have a cardiovascular condition, the importance of consistency cannot be overemphasized. Sporadic exercise can exacerbate existing coronary problems and can even bring on a heart attack. Alternatively, regular physical activity provides excellent protection against exercise-induced complications; individuals who frequently exercise have little if any increase in their risk of heart attack during strenuous activity. Clearly, from an exercise perspective, the best defense against a cardiac event is dedication.

At sixty-two years old, Teresa was a walking time bomb. The extent of her cardiac risk factors sounded like something out of a medical textbook: She had emphysema (due to years of heavy smoking), moderate hypertension, extremely high cholesterol, and the beginnings of adult-onset diabetes. Two years earlier, she had suffered a heart attack requiring emergency triple-bypass surgery. When discussing Teresa's exercise program, her physician stated to me in no uncertain terms, "If this woman doesn't change her lifestyle immediately, her odds of long-term survival are grim."

Teresa had to proceed very slowly with exercise. At first, she could not even endure more than five minutes of light cardiovascular activity before she would become fatigued and out of breath. But Teresa was persistent, gradually building up her strength and stamina. This latest exam had frightened her, and she was determined to make some changes. She never missed a workout.

Three years later, Teresa is a new woman. She has long since given up smoking and maintains a dedicated fitness regimen. All her cardiac symptoms have improved, and she was even able to discontinue her antihypertensive medication. Moreover, Teresa recently fulfilled a lifelong dream: She walked the New York City Marathon and finished the entire event!

CHAPTER 3

Bone Up Your Body

There are more than two hundred bones in the human body. From the large femur in your thigh to the tiny phalanges in your fingers, bones are multipurpose entities. They provide structural support for muscles, protect vital organs from injury, facilitate the production of red blood cells, and act as a storage site for calcium. They even contain a region of yellow bone marrow that stores fat cells, providing a long-term energy reserve for periods of extreme starvation.

But contrary to popular belief, bones aren't dormant, inanimate objects; rather, they are living, growing tissue with blood vessels and nerves, much like the kidneys, heart, and muscles. From a physiologic perspective, bones are composed of a supporting network of tissue called extracellular matrix—a composite of about 25 percent water, 25 percent collagen, and 50 percent mineral salts (including calcium phosphate, calcium carbonate, and small amounts of fluoride and magnesium). In combination, these components serve to make bones the hardest, most durable substance in the human body. When healthy, they are strong enough to resist in excess of 25,000 pounds per square inch of compression and 15,000 pounds per square inch of tension!

There are two types of bone: cortical and trabecular. Cortical bone is made up of a dense, opaque material that is extremely tough and resilient and primarily comprises the exterior portion of bone.

Because of its ability to provide a great degree of stiffness and strength in a relatively compact structure, cortical bone is best able to withstand high-tensile forces.

Trabecular bone, on the other hand, is considerably more complex than cortical bone. It lines the walls of the interior portion of bone and is made up of a spongy material that has an intricate network of rods and plates, resembling the crisscross pattern of cables on a bridge. This interconnecting structure allows trabecular bone to adapt to the extent of a load in such a way as to maximize strength while minimizing weight.

An important aspect of bone is its vast labyrinth of channels called Haversian canals. There are hundreds of these canals interspersed throughout the inside of every bone, and they serve a very important purpose: Blood vessels within the canals carry nutrients and oxygen to the bone cells and remove any accumulated waste products (such as ammonia and carbon dioxide) from circulation. In this way, bone cells receive proper nourishment so they can remain healthy and strong.

REMODELING

Like all living tissues, bone cells are constantly dying off. The body deals with this event through a process called *remodeling*. Simply stated, remodeling is the ongoing procedure of breaking down and building up of bone tissue in order to maintain optimal function. The entire remodeling cycle takes about four months to complete and continues throughout the course of your life.

Remodeling begins with bone resorption. To accomplish resorption, your body produces cells called osteoclasts whose job is to break down old bone tissue. Osteoclasts attach themselves to the extracellular matrix and hollow out microscopic areas of bone. Think of them as a demolition team, excavating unneeded materials so that renovation can take place.

Once osteoclasts have done their job, bone formation commences. Here, protein-secreting cells called osteoblasts are activated, which are responsible for laying down new bone. They patch up the holes left by the osteoclasts and rebuild bone tissue. Under ideal circumstances, the new bone is as strong—or even stronger—than the old.

BONE AND AGING

During adolescence, bone formation tends to be greater than breakdown. The activity of osteoblasts far exceeds that of osteoclasts, allowing new bone tissue to be added to the skeleton at a healthy rate. Increases in bone mineral density continue throughout the third decade of life, and generally peak at around thirty years of age.

After the age of thirty, though, things begin to turn around. Osteoblasts become less efficient at making new bone tissue, and consequently bone is stripped away faster than it is replaced. This brings about a condition called osteopenia (bone loss) which, unless counteracted by proper exercise and nutrition, only gets worse as time goes by.

The loss of bone is exacerbated by a sedentary lifestyle. You see, the cells of bone are very sensitive to weight-bearing activity. If there is not a perceived need to withstand loads, bone has no impetus to regenerate and osteopenia worsens. The most dramatic examples of this are seen in astronauts during space travel. Significant bone demineralization has been noted in these subjects after only a brief period of weightlessness. Albeit to a lesser degree, these same alterations in bone mineral density become evident in people who are very inactive.

OSTEOPOROSIS

In some cases, osteopenia can become so severe that it degenerates into osteoporosis, a debilitating disease that affects some twenty million Americans. Literally, osteoporosis translates into "porous bone" (*osteo* means bone; *porosis* means porous). It is characterized by a structural deterioration of bone mineral density, leading to bone fragility and an increased susceptibility to fractures. As the disease progresses, bones become so brittle that they can break from ordinary daily activities. A bend, a slip, or even a mere cough or sneeze is enough to snap a bone in two. Those afflicted become so frail that family members are sometimes afraid to give them a hug for fear of causing injury.

Due to its propensity to strike without warning, osteoporosis is often referred to as the "silent killer." A person can feel perfectly fit and healthy, with no telltale symptoms, and then . . . disaster occurs. Only after a crushing fall or enfeebling back injury is the condition accurately diagnosed.

One of the most common sites of osteoporosis is at the spine. With spinal osteoporosis, there is a dramatic loss of bone in the vertebral column, which leads to a diminished physical stature. Perhaps you've heard that people "get shorter" as they get older. Well, this isn't due to age per se, but rather to a squashing of the vertebrae from the weight of the body. The effects here can be quite noticeable. Depending on its severity, spinal osteoporosis can result in a loss of as much as six inches in height!

Spinal osteoporosis also has a negative effect on posture. Early on, it causes stooped shoulders, contributing to a tired, haggard-looking appearance. In advanced stages of the disease, there is a gross distortion of the spine's normal curves. This leads to the development of a *dowager's hump*—an exaggerated protrusion in the upper back and a shortening of the chest area. The compression of the chest and abdominal regions limits the ability of the lungs to expand during inspiration. Consequently, the heart can't deliver blood to the lungs efficiently, reducing the body's cardiovascular capacity and, in severe cases, causing heart failure (called *cor pulmonale*).

The other common site of osteoporosis is at the hip—a condition that often leads to hip fracture. Make no mistake: The ramifications of a hip fracture can be devastating. Hundreds of thousands are hospitalized each year due to this malady, and roughly half of them never recover from the incident. They end up spending the rest of their days convalescing in a nursing home or chronic-care facility.

Bedridden and unable to care for themselves, they inevitably develop other, more serious complications. Sadly, almost 25 percent of these victims die within a year's time.

All too often, women are oblivious to the prospect of a hip fracture. They are much more likely to fear cancer of the breast or reproductive organs. Realize, though, that a woman's lifetime risk of hip fracture alone is equal to her combined risk of developing breast, uterine, and ovarian cancer! What's more, the incidence of hip fracture increases exponentially with age, rising to almost 20 percent of all women over sixty-five.

A WOMAN'S PROBLEM

Comprising approximately 80 percent of all reported cases, women are particularly susceptible to osteoporosis. The primary culprit here is estrogen. Besides its role as a female sex hormone, estrogen is responsible for a host of regulatory functions, including the preservation of bone mineral density. Estrogen is believed to exert its effects by inhibiting bone resorption rather than by promoting new bone mineral formation.

Because estrogen has an osteo-protective effect, women are somewhat safeguarded in their premenopausal years. Accordingly, bone loss is rather modest between the ages of thirty and fifty, averaging less than ½ percent per year. The problem arises when a woman reaches menopause. During this period, there is a profound decrease in estrogen production. And without the osteogenic (bone-building) properties of estrogen, bone mineral density rapidly deteriorates. During the first five years after menopause, bone loss can be as high as 3 percent. Every year thereafter, the rate of loss

June was a frail, forty-six-year-old woman who came to me with one goal: to improve her bone density. In a recent physical exam, her physician performed a routine bone scan that showed a slight reduction in her skeletal mass. Because of her history, June's physician stated that she was at serious risk of developing osteoporosis and had to do something about it immediately.

June had all the risk factors for bone disease: She had experienced a premature menopause, with an onset at age forty-one. She was sedentary and had a family history of osteoporosis (her grandmother died after breaking her hip in an injury related to this disease). June, however, was committed to avoiding this fate.

Although there were several contraindications for exercise, I was able to put June on a regimented training program. She began to work out religiously, and her strength quickly improved. After one year, June went back for another bone scan: She had regained almost 6 percent of the density that was lost!

slows down to an extent, but is still increased above premenopausal levels at an annual rate of about 1 percent.

But menopause isn't the only estrogen-related factor in osteoporosis. Other afflictions that bring about menstrual dysfunction (such as anorexia nervosa, overtraining syndrome, etc.) also can hasten the onset of the disease. These anomalies disrupt normal estrogen balance, causing bone resorption similar to that seen during menopause. Consequently, osteoporosis isn't just an old ladies' disease—it can manifest in women as young as their late teens or early twenties.

THE LOOK GREAT AT ANY AGE PRESCRIPTION

Fortunately, if you follow the Look Great at Any Age program, bone loss doesn't have to be a natural part of aging. Time and again, exercise has clearly proven to offset the age-related decline in bone mineral density. It not only helps to maintain existing bone mass, but also can improve the strength of your bones. Gains of over 5 percent in bone mineral density have been noted in less than a year of regimented training. In postmenopausal women, these results are comparable to, or better than, hormone-replacement therapy, without any of the potential side effects!

But it's important to realize that when it comes to combating bone loss, not all types of exercise are alike. In order to build new bone tissue, the exercise must be of weight-bearing nature. Hence, some of the popular aerobic activities such as riding a stationary bike or using an elliptical machine will have virtually no effect on preventing bone loss. Other modalities like jogging, running, and/or stair climbing are only slightly better in this regard. Because results are regionally specific to the areas trained, these activities mainly target bone mineral density in the lower extremities; the spine and upper body receive little or no benefit. What's more, since these activities are performed at submaximal intensity, any bone-building effects are modest, at best.

The Look Great at Any Age program is specifically designed to build up your bones. Because of the intense, weight-bearing nature of the routine, bone is sufficiently stimulated to strengthen itself. You see, bone cells are sensitive to load-induced strain. When loads are continuously applied to the skeletal system, there is an adaptive response causing increases in bone mineral density. This is the body's way of avoiding future bone-related damage. New bone formation occurs from the tension associated with the contraction of muscle at the point where it attaches to bone. This is accomplished both by decreased bone resorption (by the inhibition of the production of osteoclasts) and increased bone formation (by the acceleration of the production of osteoblasts). It is hypothesized that an increased amount of blood flow to the Haversian canals improves bone-related nutrient utilization and therefore contributes to the process.

One of the most visible effects of the program is its positive impact on posture. You will begin to stand taller, projecting a youthful exuberance. Any distortion in the normal curvature of your spine will gradually be reversed. The upshot of this physical transformation will transcend into every facet of your life. You'll display an aura of self-confidence that commands respect both in professional and social endeavors.

An additional benefit of the program is that it helps to improve balance. A loss of balance heightens the possibility of falling, which has been implicated in a majority of the cases of hip fractures. Since motor skills tend to deteriorate with age, this is especially important as you get older. By consistently adhering to the exercise routine, you'll "wake up" nerve impulses that control muscles, thereby improving your functional capacity. The effect on wellness is dramatic: Studies have conclusively shown that physically active individuals cut their risk of hip fracture in half when compared to those who are sedentary.

From a bone-building perspective, the earlier you start the Look Great at Any Age program the better. It has been shown that starting an exercise routine in your teens or early twenties can stave off the ravages of osteoporosis. Since bone formation is greatest during adolescence, it's important to try to build up your bones when you are young. Doing so creates a "bone bank" that provides a reserve for later in life. Think of it like a retirement account: If you accumulate a large nest egg, you can live comfortably throughout your golden years, but if your savings are meager, you'll soon go bankrupt.

That said, you can still derive excellent bone-building benefits from the program even if you are a senior citizen; regimented weight training has been shown to significantly improve functional mobility in frail nursing home patients up to ninety-six years of age! The message is clear: No matter how old you are, it's never too late to exercise!

CHAPTER 4

Work Out the Blues

I n today's fast-paced society, stress is literally everywhere. Deadlines, rush-hour traffic, inflation . . . the list of stressors goes on and on. Whether it's at home or on the job, there simply is no escape from the daily grind of life's travails.

By definition, stress is the physical and emotional strain on your body in response to the demands of daily living. It can arise from a plethora of factors, including work issues, interpersonal dealings, and the environment.

But stress isn't always a bad thing. In fact, when stress is properly channeled, it can be a positive influence. The birth of a child, a job promotion, and a new relationship are examples of stressful events that have the potential of bringing about great joy and happiness. If you have the right mindset, these events can result in an exciting new perspective on life, pushing you to be your best.

All too often, however, stress is not properly managed and builds up over time. Chronic stress, which results from repeated exposure to stress for a period of several weeks, invariably becomes a negative influence. The primary offender here is the hormone cortisol. Cortisol is released from your adrenal glands in response to a stressful event and serves to raise heart rate and blood pressure, as well as diverting blood sugar from the internal organs to the brain.

If stress is only transient, your body is resilient enough to deal with a surge in cortisol without ill effect. But when cortisol levels remain elevated for prolonged periods, bad things are bound to happen. For one, there is a suppression of lymphocytes—a class of white blood cells that are essential for proper immune function. This weakens your immune system resulting in an increased predisposition to colds, infections, and influenza, as well as a greater sensitivity to allergens.

Persistent secretion of cortisol also has a negative impact on your body. You see, cortisol is catabolic—it breaks down bodily tissues—and one of its targets is muscle. When cortisol levels are abnormally high, there is a breakdown of muscle protein, which results in a release of amino acids (the "building blocks" of protein) into the bloodstream. These amino acids are then used to synthesize glucose (by a process called *gluconeogenesis)* to fuel the brain so that it can maintain a heightened state of alertness. But this phenomenon is clearly a double-edged sword: Precious muscle tone is lost, thereby diminishing the quality of your physique.

Early symptoms of negative stress include headaches, back pain, and neck and shoulder discomfort. If the stress is allowed to linger on, complications can become serious: Altered sugar metabolism can worsen diabetes; increased gastric acidity can aggravate ulcers; and persistently increased cardiac output and constriction of blood vessels can contribute to the development of coronary artery disease. All things considered, recurrent stress is not something to be taken lightly.

DEPRESSION

Under certain conditions, stress can lead to depression—a brain disorder that impairs the body's biological capacity to create and balance a normal range of thoughts and emotions. A serious loss, personal illness, financial crisis, or other exceedingly stressful situations can overwhelm a person, ultimately triggering a depressive event. If left untreated, symptoms can last for weeks, months, or even years.

Unlike some other diseases, depression is not an "all-or-nothing" phenomenon. Rather, there are different degrees of the disease, and the severity varies greatly from person to person. Three broad classifications of depression have been identified:

- *Depressed mood:* This is the mildest form of depression. It is characterized by a "gloom and doom" outlook with feelings of sadness and emptiness. Although often temporary, it can sometimes progress into more severe depressive states.
- *Dysthymia:* This chronic, low-grade form of depression is characterized by low self-esteem and persistent dejection. It is accompanied by changes in energy levels, appetite, and/or sleeping patterns and impairs a person's ability to function in everyday life.
- *Major depression:* This is the most severe form of depression. It is characterized by persistent despondency, with a complete loss of interest in normal daily activities. Symptoms include decreased energy levels, sleep disturbances, loss of appetite, and feelings of utter hopelessness. For many, it is so incapacitating that they cannot even get out of bed. In the most severe cases, psychotic symptoms and/or suicidal tendencies predominate.

Because of the negative stigma attached to the disease, depression frequently goes undiagnosed; some people are simply too embarrassed to confront the problem and seek treatment. As much as one-fifth of the population will, at some time in their lives, experience a depressive event, and approximately 8 percent will suffer from major depression. Given that the World Health Organization ranks depression as the world's fourth most devastating illness, the ramifications in terms of public health are enormous.

The underlying cause of depression is most often related to low serotonin levels. Serotonin is part of a class of compounds known as *neurotransmitters* whose principal job is to carry vital signals between certain brain cells. For the brain to function properly, it must have balanced levels of serotonin—a lack of it invariably leads to mood disturbance.

Depression in Women

On average, women are approximately twice as likely to suffer from depression as their male counterparts. This is partly attributable to their myriad responsibilities. In addition to the traditional chores of tending to the house and kids, many women now hold down full-time jobs. After spending a hard day at work, they have to go shopping, get food on the table, take care of the children, and perform a host of other domestic tasks. Over time, these diverse obligations can become overly burdensome, seriously taxing a woman's ability to cope with stresses.

Monthly hormonal fluctuations also appear to play a role in female depression. It has been well documented that serotonin levels become suppressed in the premenstrual period. This sudden and precipitous drop in serotonin is considered to be the genesis of symptoms associated with premenstrual syndrome (PMS). Depending on a woman's mental state, mood disturbance can transcend the monthly cycle and carry over into daily life.

Pregnancy is another contributing factor to mental illness. While hormonal irregularities appear to play a role here, the changes in body composition are equally contributory. During term, a woman undergoes many physiologic changes that significantly alter her physique. Certain areas expand, others stretch, and still others sag due to the demands of carrying a child. It is commonplace to gain thirty, forty, or even fifty pounds during pregnancy. For some, this causes a loss of self-esteem that ultimately leads to a depressed state.

Women are particularly prone to bouts of depression after delivery. Despite good intentions, some simply aren't prepared to care for another human being. The extreme change in lifestyle associated with childbirth is sometimes too much to bear and can set off a full-blown depressive event. This illness, commonly termed *postpartum depression,* affects as many as 14 percent of new mothers. Occasionally, it can lead to *postpartum psychosis,* a disease characterized by hallucinations and delusions about the baby. Needless to say, the consequences of this condition can be disastrous.

Depression and Aging

More than any other demographic group, the elderly are prone to mental illness. The realization that one is entering the twilight of life is a scary thought that often brings about a great deal of soul-searching. What's more, the numerous stresses associated with aging (including health concerns, retirement issues, and family problems) increase the mental burden, heightening the potential of falling into a depression.

For women, the age-related onset of depression is often attributed to menopause but it is still being debated whether or not the disease is related to hormonal changes seen during this period. Menopause is accompanied by a host of mental and physical complications such as hot flashes, night sweats, and vaginal dryness, which certainly can contribute to emotional distress. What's more, there is some evidence that the low estrogen production associated with menopause correlates with a decrease in serotonin levels—a major risk-factor in mental illness. Despite these parallels, however, a clear cause-and-effect relationship between menopause and depression has yet to be established.

More likely, the link between mental health and menopause is related to a woman's attitude toward the phenomenon. It is known that traumatic changes in life patterns can trigger a depressive episode and, to some, menopause is quite traumatic. The reduced estrogen production causes a shift in body contour as many women gain weight through their abdomens; there is a deepening of the voice, an increase in unwanted body hair, and a loss of fertility. In sum, many of the qualities associated with womanhood are altered, which can lead to feelings of inadequacy and, thereby, anxiety.

THE LOOK GREAT AT ANY AGE PRESCRIPTION

The Look Great at Any Age program is designed to have a positive impact on mental health—not only in treatment, but also in prevention. The demanding nature of the program is, in itself, a de-stressor. As you work out, your mind must be focused to perform the task at hand. Worries about work, family, or anything else, for that matter, become secondary. There's simply no opportunity to dwell on negative thoughts during training and any feelings of pent-up frustration, anger, or hostility are channeled into the weights.

What's more, there is an elevation in levels of beta-endorphins—a group of opiatelike compounds that help to promote pleasure and reduce pain. Endorphins are extremely powerful, having more than one hundred times the potency of morphine. As you exercise, these chemicals are released from the pituitary gland and into the bloodstream, where they attach to brain "receptors" and generate a feeling of euphoria often referred to as an "exercise high." One of the reasons that exercise becomes addicting after a while is that you simply feel better about yourself after training.

For those with depression, the program can be especially beneficial. In the past, traditional forms of antidepressive treatment were limited to psychotherapy and medication. Although these remedies can be reasonably effective forms of treatment, they pose a tremendous financial burden to the patient and the health-care system. According to the President's Council on Physical Fitness, depressed individuals spend over 50 percent more on health care than those who are not depressed. Further, those being treated with antidepressants spend three times as much on outpatient pharmacy costs as those not on drug therapy.

There is also a distinct risk of negative side effects associated with antidepressant medication. Even the newer drugs such as Prozac and Zoloft, which are supposedly safer than previous medications, carry the potential for adverse reactions (including weight gain, drowsiness, and sexual dysfunction). So while drug therapy has its place in treating mental illness, it is by no means a panacea.

Fortunately, the Look Great at Any Age program provides an excellent alternative to drug therapy, helping to relieve symptoms of depression and anxiety as well as improving overall mood. It is now irrefutable that a definitive relationship exists between physical fitness and mental health. Provided that the routine is performed on a regular, consistent basis, it is often at least as effective as medication in combating depression. Better yet, results can be seen in a matter of weeks—all without side effects!

Antidepressive benefits are achieved, in part, by increasing the uptake of serotonin in the brain.

Betty approached my office with a great deal of trepidation. "This isn't going to work," she said. "I've tried virtually everything, and I don't see how a personal trainer can help me any more than my psychiatrist!"

Betty, a slender fifty-two-year-old, had been suffering from clinical depression for the past eight years and had been undergoing intensive psychotherapy throughout this time. She had taken a variety of different prescription medications and had even tried several herbal remedies to cure her illness. Although her condition had improved, she still endured periods of severe despondency. She recently began seeing a new psychiatrist who recommended that she try exercise to supplement her therapy . . .

At first, Betty was quite resistant to exercise and objected to virtually everything in the program. However, she gradually began to embrace her workouts and started to see results. Her energy levels increased, she gained strength, and she even developed a pretty fair degree of muscle tone. Little by little, her self-esteem improved with an appreciable effect on her persona.

After three months of working out, Betty was a fine testament to the efficacy of exercise as an antidepressant. In fact, after a recent session she happily remarked, "Everyone keeps telling me how cheerful I seem lately. Even my husband says he's noticed a big difference—and that's really saying something!"

This is accomplished by boosting levels of free tryptophan—an essential amino acid that acts as a precursor to serotonin. As you train, the breakdown of fat separates tryptophan from a transport protein called albumin. Since albumin cannot cross the blood brain barrier (a wall of vessels that buffers certain compounds from entering the brain), the amount of tryptophan that can be used for production of serotonin becomes limited. When tryptophan is freed from albumin, circulating levels of the amino acid are significantly increased, allowing it to readily traverse the blood brain barrier and be used for serotonin synthesis.

Additional benefits are realized by helping to regulate sleeping patterns. It has been well-documented that stress and depression often cause insomnia and various other sleep disturbances. These, in turn, can exacerbate mood disturbances and irritability. By signaling the body to rest, exercise actually induces sleep. After adapting to the program, you'll to tend to fall asleep more quickly and have a deeper, more restful sleep. Ultimately, this can have a positive impact on enhancing your state of mind and alleviating depressive symptoms.

Perhaps the most important way that the program counteracts depression is by improving self-esteem. This is accomplished on multiple levels. For one, it has been shown that when a depressed individual becomes motivated enough to exercise, her self-esteem is raised and, in turn, depression lessens. Moreover, exercise can help a person achieve a feeling of control over her life, giving her a sense of mastery and thereby improving mood. And, of course, the positive change in appearance associated with exercise is extremely uplifting. As the old saying goes, "When you look good, you feel good." By simply improving body composition, a huge difference can be seen in state of mind.

THE
FITNESS
SOLUTION

PART TWO

CHAPTER 5

Before You Begin

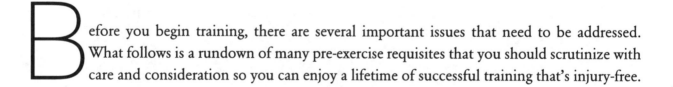

Before you begin training, there are several important issues that need to be addressed. What follows is a rundown of many pre-exercise requisites that you should scrutinize with care and consideration so you can enjoy a lifetime of successful training that's injury-free.

MEDICAL CHECKUP

Prior to commencing the Look Great at Any Age program, it is beneficial to visit your physician and get a complete medical checkup. If you are over the age of fifty, a checkup should be considered mandatory. This will ensure that you are physically ready to engage in vigorous exercise and rule out potential training-related contraindications.

A checkup generally consists of a medical screen (including questions about prior health, family history, medications taken, and others), a battery of blood tests, a bone-density exam, and an exercise-tolerance test that monitors your heart, lungs, and blood-oxygen levels while riding a stationary bike or jogging on a treadmill. Together, the results will give your physician a snapshot of your current physical status and provide a solid basis for determining any possible contraindications for exercise.

If it is found that you have a medical condition that contraindicates exercise, give this book to your physician and ask him specifically what you can and cannot do. Virtually everyone is capable of working out. When properly administered, physical activity has proven to be a safe, effective remedy for improving the health and fitness of those with conditions as diverse as congestive heart failure, coronary artery disease, osteoarthritis, peripheral vascular disease, and many other anomalies. Regardless of your medical status, chances are that you should be able to undertake this program, albeit with certain limitations.

SAFETY PRECAUTIONS

Even if you are given the go-ahead to exercise without restrictions, it doesn't necessarily mean that you are in the clear. If you are afflicted with any of a variety of disorders, certain precautionary measures must be taken while you're working out. Below are some of the more common medical conditions along with their corresponding safety procedures; follow them as directed.

IF YOU HAVE DIABETES:
- Consume a meal approximately one to two hours before training.
- Check your blood-glucose level before training; if it is above 250 mg/dl or below 100 mg/dl, refrain from exercise.
- Keep a supply of simple carbohydrates (such as a bagel, juice, fruit, or sports drink) around in case of a hypoglycemic event.

IF YOU HAVE ARTHRITIS:
- Modify any exercise that causes you discomfort.
- Avoid gripping the weights too tightly.
- If joint pain lasts longer than two hours postworkout, ease up on the intensity of training in your next session.
- If joint pain significantly interferes with your exercise ability, consult your physician about taking pain relievers.

IF YOU HAVE HYPERTENSION:
- Avoid gripping the weights too tightly.
- Make sure you never hold your breath during training.
- Check your blood pressure before exercise; if the reading is greater than 160/100, refrain from training.

On a general level, if you experience any adverse symptoms during a workout (such as nausea, headache, dizziness, or pain), stop training immediately. If the symptoms persist, visit your physician so he or she can determine their origin. Something that may seem like a minor nuisance can be the precursor of a serious health problem.

EQUIPMENT NEEDED

Okay, you've received medical clearance to begin the Look Great at Any Age program. So where do you go from here? Well, you now need to purchase the equipment necessary to perform the routine.

Fortunately, this program is designed to be performed in the comfort of your own home with a minimal amount of exercise paraphernalia. The following is a list of what is required:

- *Dumbbells:* Dumbbells are the primary tools in your training arsenal. You will need a set of two-, three-, five-, eight-, and ten-pound dumbbells to start. Depending on your strength levels, additional dumbbells will be necessary as your strength increases.
- *Leg Weights:* Ankle weights provide increased resistance for body-weight movements. Get ones that can accommodate ten-pound weight insertions. Depending on your strength levels, a second set may be necessary.
- *Bench:* An adjustable weight bench is an indispensable component of any home gym. It allows you to train at various degrees of incline and decline, affording the ability to vary your movements and hit your muscles from different angles. Make sure you buy one that's sturdy; you don't want it to give out while you're in the middle of a set!

WHAT TO WEAR, WHERE TO TRAIN

Women generally put a great deal of thought into their attire—and working out is no exception. There is a whole industry specifically devoted to workout gear. Designer exercise clothing is a billion-dollar business, with certain outfits costing upwards of several hundred dollars.

In reality, though, it makes little difference what you wear during training. The most expensive workout clothes won't make you perform any better than an old pair of sweats. It is best to wear any type of clothing that makes you feel comfortable. As a rule, loose-fitting attire is best; it lets you move about more freely and allows rapid dissipation of body heat.

Footwear is probably the most important clothing-related consideration for exercise. A good pair of sneakers is a must. Make sure you get shoes that provide good support and protection. Important features include a strong, stable heel, good arch support, a comfortable insole, and a durable, cushioned outsole. Cross-training sneakers are generally a good all-around choice, but many other fitness sneakers are also satisfactory. Never wear sandals or open-toed shoes during exercise—they are dangerous when training and can easily contribute to an injury.

In setting up your home gym, make sure that the area is relatively cool, but not too cold. An overly hot and/or humid training environment can lead to heat-related illness or even heatstroke. On the other hand, an extremely cold environment prevents your muscles and joints from functioning properly. Performance is compromised, and the potential for a connective tissue injury is heightened.

WARM-UP

Before training, it is important to perform a brief warm-up. The purpose of the warm-up is to thoroughly ready your body for vigorous exercise. Not only does it diminish the possibility of sustaining an injury, but it also helps to increase range of motion, improve muscular responsiveness, and speed up recovery. Regardless of your level of experience, the warm-up should remain simple and straightforward. Since the intent is to prepare yourself for intense training, not to challenge your resources, advanced techniques and fancy maneuvers are superfluous. Chapter 6 will discuss warming up in detail.

THE FITNESS LIFESTYLE

Finally, it's important to realize that there isn't a quick fix for improving your appearance and health; for lasting benefits, fitness must become a way of life. But, if you implement the program on a regular, consistent basis, you should be able to realize tangible results in a fairly short period of time. Within the first month, you should see substantial changes in your strength and endurance, with increased energy and reduced stress. You'll notice that your clothes fit a little better and that you are firmer in places that were once flabby. Over the next several months, these improvements will magnify, producing significant progress in both body composition and health. Live the fitness lifestyle and you'll change your life forever!

CHAPTER 6

Pump Up Your Fitness

For many women, weight training can be downright scary. After all, lifting a heavy, inanimate object is a chore that most try to avoid. On initial consultation, I've actually had women tell me they'd rather endure dental surgery than lift weights! If you are one who is intimidated by the mere thought of strenuous activity, don't fret. To paraphrase Franklin Delano Roosevelt, "You have nothing to fear but fear itself."

This routine is specifically designed for those who are averse to weight training. It takes into account all levels of strength and ability. The easy-to-understand step-by-step format gives you all the tools you will need for long-term success on a strength-training program.

The Look Great at Any Age program incorporates weight training into an aerobic format, helping to promote muscular as well as cardiorespiratory fitness. Both of these factors are integral components of overall health that enhance your physical and mental well-being. In short order, you will increase your strength, improve your posture, reduce your body fat, tone your muscles, and improve your bone density. Along the way, you will develop a strong, shapely physique—one that exudes confidence and femininity.

It is important to note that this is *not* a body-sculpting routine, per se. While the shape of your body certainly will change dramatically over time, you shouldn't expect to win a physique contest from your training efforts. Body sculpting is a complex process requiring a more elaborate and intensive routine—one that includes multiple sets and advanced training techniques. If, at some point, you should decide to pursue this lofty ambition, you can consult my book *Sculpting Her Body Perfect* (Human Kinetics Publishers). It comprehensively details a system of training that will help you sculpt your body to its genetic potential.

However, assuming that your goal is to achieve a lean, toned, aesthetically pleasing physique, you should be ecstatic with the results obtained from this routine. It will make you look and feel great, taking your body far beyond where you might previously have believed possible. You will notice muscles that you never knew you had, and you will be able to easily perform chores that in the past seemed laborious. You will have better self-esteem, increased energy reserves, and reduced levels of stress. In sum, you will be well on your way to achieving the ultimate objective of this program: looking and feeling great, no matter what your age.

I will begin by discussing the intricacies of this routine, expounding the theory behind the exercises, reps and sets, and intensity levels required for performance. No stone is left unturned, putting you on the cutting edge of training science. Don't worry, though: The information will be covered in a user-friendly manner, and the technical jargon will be kept to a bare minimum.

Finally, a sample routine is outlined, providing a three-day workout. Each exercise is explained in detail with descriptive photos showing the start and finish positions of the movements. In order to help you with technique, expert training tips are supplied that highlight the nuances of exercise performance.

WARMING UP

So you're ready to start training, right? Well, not quite so fast . . .

Before each workout, you must perform a general warm-up. Although you might be tempted to save time by forgoing the warm-up, this would be a mistake. Doing so only serves to jeopardize your well-being, putting your body and health in danger.

The purpose of the warm-up is to elevate your core temperature and increase blood flow throughout your body. There is a direct correlation between muscle temperature and exercise performance: The higher a muscle's temperature (within a safe range), the better its ability to contract. Simply stated, a muscle can produce more force when it is sufficiently warmed up, which ultimately leads to a better workout. What's more, by elevating core temperature, you reduce the amount of friction in your joints. The net effect is an increase in range of motion and improved joint-related resiliency.

An excellent way to begin the general warm-up is with a period of light cardiovascular exercise. Virtually any cardiovascular activity can be used including the stationary bike, stair climber, treadmill, jumping rope—the choice is up to you. Some people enjoy performing a variety of different activities to reduce boredom, while others prefer to keep their warm-up constant. Either way is fine, as long as the basic objective is met.

Your warm-up activity should be performed at a relatively low level of intensity, continuing only until you have broken a light sweat. Your heart rate should be approximately 50 percent of your maximum heart rate (220 minus your age). Adjust the intensity of your warm-up as needed to keep a steady, even tempo, and concentrate on maintaining a stable pulse. You should not feel tired or out of breath either during or after performance. Your goal during warm-up is merely to warm your body tissues and accelerate blood flow—not to achieve cardiovascular benefits or reduce body fat. Consequently, if you are at all fatigued from your efforts, then you are training too hard. If so, reduce the pace of exercise and proceed in a more relaxed fashion.

One notion currently accepted as gospel in many fitness circles is that you must stretch before a workout. The popular belief is that pre-exercise stretching helps to prevent training-related injuries. The truth is, however, that stretching before exercise does little to prevent injuries. You can stretch all you want before training, but it won't diminish the chances of pulling a muscle or damaging connective tissue. Now this isn't to say that staying flexible is unimportant with respect to injury. On the contrary, it certainly is. Studies have shown that there is a correlation between poor joint mobility and an increased incidence of exercise-related injuries: a fact that is offset by flexibility training. Realize, though, that stretching does not necessarily have to be part of a warm-up in order to deliver benefits—it can be done at any time, whether it's before, during, or after your workout.

In final analysis, if you choose to stretch before exercise, do so to improve flexibility—not to stave off injury. While stretching is certainly a beneficial activity, it really doesn't matter *when* the stretching is performed from a preventative standpoint. As long as you incorporate regular flexibility training into your routine, it can be done before, during or after a workout. It even can be done on your rest days as stretching shouldn't have any negative impact on recovery. The important thing is to maintain good mobility in the joints, allowing them to execute full range moves without restraint.

Your warm-up, not including any stretching, should last about five minutes or so—any more is unnecessary. Upon completion, you're now prepared to work out.

EXERCISES

As you probably know, there is a plethora of exercises from which to choose, each one targeting a specific area of your body. Many of these movements can be adapted to free weights, cables, machines, and other pieces of equipment, creating an endless array of possibilities. With so many choices available, it is easy for a beginner to become overwhelmed with options.

In order to minimize confusion, routines in this book keep things simple. Chapters 7, 8, and 9 outline three distinct exercise routines that can be performed at home—no gym is required (although you certainly can use a gym if desired). During the first few months of training, you should do the same exercises each time you work out so that you become comfortable with the lifting process without the worry of learning new movements. As time progresses, the routine will become more dynamic so that you will advance in conjunction with your progress. When you are ready, new exercises should be introduced in order to further your development. You can find a list of additional movements on my website at www.lookgreatnaked.com/resources//descriptions/descriptions.htm.

Motor Skills

One of the most intimidating aspects of weight training is the initial awkwardness while performing the exercises. It is normal for anyone to feel grossly uncoordinated when she first attempts to lift weights. Unlike most cardiovascular activities such as walking, biking, and stair climbing, weight training utilizes movements that are not practical to everyday life. When are you ever required to lift an object in a controlled fashion over a precise range of motion, using certain muscles to the exclusion of others? Probably never, which can make your first few workouts arduous, frustrating endeavors.

The good news is that with proper diligence and a little patience, lifting weights soon becomes second nature. Through repetition, your muscles quickly learn the necessary motor skills for weight training. Within a brief period of time, you will be able to execute each movement in perfect form, looking like a pro.

Regardless of your athletic prowess, there undoubtedly will be certain exercises that continually give you difficulty. Most likely, these movements simply are not suited to your body type. For instance, taller people tend to have a more difficult time performing squats because of the long range of motion required. You should, therefore, consider your own body characteristics when choosing movements to include in your workout. If you are not comfortable with an exercise, simply substitute a complementary maneuver that works the same muscle group. Ultimately, you should choose only exercises that best accentuate your own body structure, discarding those that prove to be a problem.

Total Body Training

It is important to take a total-body approach to training, working each major muscle group into play every time you exercise. Through this weight-training program, your chest, upper back, shoulders, biceps, triceps, quads, hams/glutes, calves, and abdominals will each be targeted during a session, ensuring complete, symmetrical development of your physique. In order to allow adequate recuperation between opposing muscle groups, it is recommended that you adhere to the prescribed order of the exercises. This will keep your muscles fresh throughout the session and heighten your muscular endurance.

Furthermore, it is essential that you follow protocol and train all your major muscle groups without exception. All too often, women selectively work the muscles they are most concerned with improving and neglect others. However, your muscles function holistically, working in concert with one another to perform everyday tasks. When one muscle is trained at the expense of another, you create structural imbalances that throw off your body's symmetry. Not only does this ruin the aesthetics of your physique, but it can also substantially increase your risk of injury.

Figures 6A and 6B show the major muscles of the human body. Make a point to learn their anatomical positions and functions; doing so will help you immeasurably in your training endeavors.

Compound Movements

Every exercise falls into one of two categories: *compound movements* or *isolation movements*. A compound movement is any exercise that incorporates more than one joint in exercise performance. For example, the flat dumbbell press (see page 60) is a compound movement since action occurs at both the shoulder and elbow joints in the completion of the lift. On the other hand, an isolation movement requires the use of only one joint in exercise performance. The triceps kickback (see page 68) is an example of this type of movement, since only the elbow joint is used during the maneuver.

In order to build a solid structural foundation, compound movements are of particular importance during the early stages of training. Because their performance involves the use of many supporting muscles (called stabilizer muscles), they are the most efficient way to exercise because they accelerate the rate at which you develop your physique. Accordingly, the routines in Part II make liberal use of these movements, implementing them whenever possible.

Compound movements also provide the added benefit of increasing your aerobic capacity. Because they use multiple muscle groups, your body must expend more energy during performance. This causes a significant elevation of your heart rate, burning up to twice as many calories as comparable isolation movements. The net effect is better cardiorespiratory fitness and improved body-fat reduction.

However, this does not diminish the significance of isolation movements. They are an excellent means of targeting specific muscles (or even specific portions of a muscle) and can help to bring lagging body parts into harmony with the rest of your physique. These types of exercises, however, are best utilized as complementary movements. In this way, you will develop a sound muscular foundation and can integrate them based on your individual needs.

Variety

Varying your use of exercises is paramount to achieving long-term success. Since your muscles readily adapt to the same exercises, repeated use of a movement will lead to decreased effectiveness. Ultimately, you will reach a plateau in your training endeavors and results will stagnate. A varied training regimen counteracts your body's adaptation response by continually keeping your muscles "off guard." Therefore, your body can never adjust to a given stimulus, thereby helping to promote ongoing improvements.

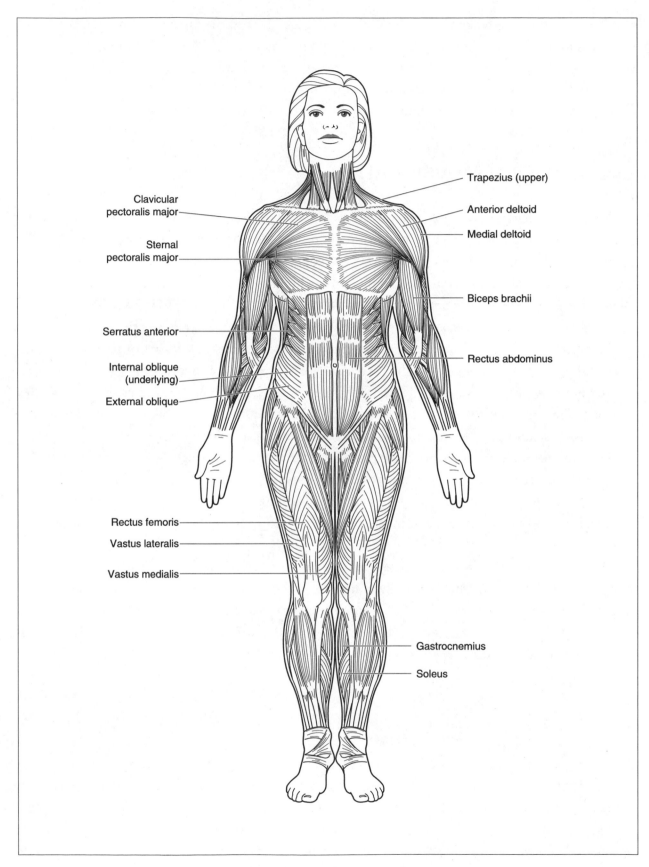

Clavicular
pectoralis major

Sternal
pectoralis major

Serratus anterior

Internal oblique
(underlying)

External oblique

Trapezius (upper)

Anterior deltoid

Medial deltoid

Biceps brachii

Rectus abdominus

Rectus femoris

Vastus lateralis

Vastus medialis

Gastrocnemius

Soleus

FIGURE 6A. FRONT VIEW OF BODY.

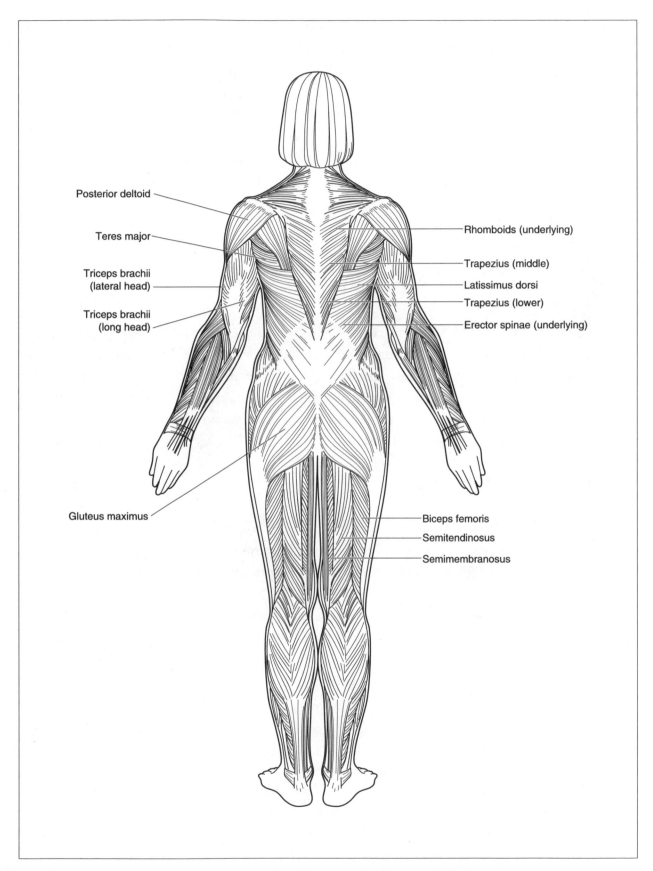

Posterior deltoid

Teres major

Triceps brachii
(lateral head)

Triceps brachii
(long head)

Gluteus maximus

Rhomboids (underlying)

Trapezius (middle)

Latissimus dorsi

Trapezius (lower)

Erector spinae (underlying)

Biceps femoris

Semitendinosus

Semimembranosus

FIGURE 6B. REAR VIEW OF BODY.

Furthermore, exercise variation allows you to work your muscles from different angles, assuring more complete muscular development. Since an exercise stimulates only a portion of the hundreds of thousands of tiny fibers that make up each muscle, the only way to target all these fibers is to employ a variety of maneuvers, each stressing your muscles in a slightly different fashion. In this way, balance and symmetry are achieved along with optimal gains in strength.

Adding variety also helps to prevent exercise boredom, which could cause you to lose interest in your routine. Each day will be a new challenge, and your motivation to train will remain high. To paraphrase an old saying; "Variety is the spice of exercise!" This is why I've provided three different routines; make sure to use them all.

REPS AND SETS

A *repetition* (or rep, for short) is one complete movement in an exercise. For instance, in the seated dumbbell curl (see page 66), when you raise the weight from your side up toward your shoulders and then return it back to the start position, you have performed a repetition. When you perform a series of reps in succession, you have performed a *set*. Reps and sets are the heart and soul of your routine, and understanding their function is essential to meeting your objectives.

High-Rep Training

You can utilize a variety of repetition ranges in order to achieve various fitness goals. While everyone has different physical and genetic limitations in terms of what she ultimately can accomplish, everyone should begin with these general rules for repetition ranges:

- A set of fifteen to twenty repetitions is best for increasing local muscular endurance. This is considered a high-repetition range and is oriented to achieving lean muscle tone.
- A set of eight to twelve repetitions is best for increasing overall muscularity. This is considered a moderate-repetition range and is oriented toward developing a bodybuilding physique.
- A set of up to six repetitions is best for increasing strength and power. This is considered a low-repetition range and is oriented to power-lifting goals.

The Look Great at Any Age routine utilizes a high-repetition format, aiming for approximately fifteen to twenty reps per set. Although some fitness professionals advocate a moderate-rep scheme, high reps provide distinct benefits for the mature woman.

Training in a high-rep fashion helps to produce an ideal complement of muscular shape and definition. The vast majority of women aren't concerned with maximizing muscular mass or power;

rather, they strive to develop a lean, toned physique. Hence, training in a low- to moderate-rep format is unnecessary and perhaps even counterproductive. Generally speaking, higher reps are more suited to the physique-oriented goals of women.

Furthermore, utilizing a high-rep scheme decreases the potential for training-related injury. Since high reps demand the use of lighter weights, less torque is placed on your joints and connective tissue, and the strain on these delicate regions is eased. And because lighter weights are also easier to control, there is a greater margin for error if a training mishap should occur.

High reps also increase the calorie-burning effects of your workout. As opposed to low reps, more of your endurance-oriented muscle fibers are targeted during high-rep training. These fibers are aerobic in nature and tend to derive their energy by burning fat for fuel. Moreover, since a high-rep set takes almost twice as long to complete as a moderate-rep set, a greater aerobic response is achieved from the exercise. The combination of these factors results in an increase in the amount of calories burned, making high reps the optimal means for fat loss.

Volume

For the purposes of this routine, you will employ only one set of one exercise per muscle group. When properly executed, a single set is all that is required to produce desired results. Unless you have body-sculpting aspirations, training in this fashion will accomplish all your fitness objectives and generate maximal results in minimal time. And, by using a low-volume approach, you will be able to maintain strength throughout your workout. As you age, you tend to fatigue more easily than before, and your energy resources become easily depleted, decreasing your ability to sustain performance levels over long periods of time. Therefore, it is essential to train in the most efficient way possible and pare down your workout to the bare necessities. As a rule, do only what you need to do—less can be more!

Mind-in-Muscle

Weight training is not merely a physical endeavor, and its mental aspect cannot be overlooked. When performing an exercise, you should consciously try to establish a *mind-to-muscle connection*. In essence, this requires visualizing the muscle that you are training and feeling that muscle work throughout each repetition. Rather than thinking about where you perceive a muscular stimulus, you must concentrate on where you are *supposed* to feel the stimulus. At first, this may seem like a foreign concept. However, until you are able to develop a mental link with your muscles, the effectiveness of your training efforts will be severely limited.

Many aspiring trainees believe that weight training is merely the action of lifting a weight from point A to point B. Unfortunately, while these individuals might perform an exercise with what appears to be satisfactory technique, they fail to adequately stimulate their target muscles. For example, in the one-arm dumbbell row (see page 62), it is quite common for a woman to feel the majority of muscular stress in her biceps and forearms. Since the biceps and forearms initiate the movement of weight in this activity, the arms will necessarily receive a good deal of stress during the lift. Hence, without applying a mind-to-muscle connection, a woman will be inclined to use her arms, rather than the target muscles of the upper back, to lift the weight. Obviously, this will diminish the overall effectiveness of the exercise.

For best results, you must consciously visualize the muscle being trained and use that muscle exclusively during exercise performance. You must be oblivious to your surroundings, with all outside distractions purged from your mind. As you perform each repetition, the target muscle must remain under continuous tension so that it is the primary mover throughout the movement.

Rep Speed

The speed at which you perform a repetition is dependent on gravity. There are two facets of a rep: the *concentric* phase and the *eccentric* phase. Due to gravitational force, each phase will dictate your speed of movement.

Concentric reps (sometimes called positives) involve lifting a weight against the force of gravity. For example, in the seated dumbbell overhead press (see page 64), this involves pressing the weight from your shoulders to the finish position. During the concentric phase, you are shortening a muscle, achieving a muscular contraction at the top of the movement. This portion of the rep should take roughly one to two seconds to complete, and your focus should be on driving through gravity with all your might.

Alternatively, eccentric reps (sometimes called negatives) move with the force of gravity. In the example of the seated dumbbell overhead press, this involves bringing the weight from the finish position back down to shoulder level. During the eccentric phase, the muscle is lengthened and stretched at the end of the movement. Your focus here should be on resisting the pull of gravity so that momentum does not take over in performance. On average, this should take about four seconds to complete, keeping tension on the muscle throughout.

The speed of your reps should be performed at a rhythmic pace. Each repetition should flow into the next, creating a distinct tempo to the set. By training in this fashion, it becomes easier to maintain concentration throughout your set and allows you to better target your muscles.

Above all, remember the ABCs of lifting: Always Be in Control. The speed at which you perform a repetition is irrelevant if you don't maintain control of the weight. As long as your reps are smooth and not dictated by momentum, you can adjust the velocity to your own level of comfort.

Breathing

It is amazing how something as natural as breathing can become such a chore during the lifting process. Proper breathing is an integral part of weight training, and its importance cannot be overstated.

Breathing should be regulated in a consistent fashion. You should begin by taking a deep breath before commencing your set. As you initiate the concentric portion of the rep, start to exhale, expelling your breath in an even manner. By the time you contract your muscle at the finish point, all your breath should be fully released. Then, on the eccentric portion of the movement, you should inhale as you return the weight to the start position, preparing yourself for the next repetition.

A good way to control breathing patterns is to count your reps out loud. As you begin the concentric portion of each rep, count in deliberate fashion: o-one, two-oo, three-ee, etc. After a while, you will automatically breathe in a regimented manner and can abandon this practice if you so choose.

Under no circumstances should you ever hold your breath while lifting! Doing so dramatically increases your blood pressure and stops blood flow back to the heart—both extremely dangerous complications, especially if you have any preexisting cardiovascular disease. Often, headaches will result (sometimes of a severe nature), and in extreme cases, you can even rupture a blood vessel in your brain.

INTENSITY

This routine uses a high-intensity program, in which you will push your muscles to exertion and train at a rapid pace. As long as you stay within your own capabilities, this type of training is perfectly safe, and will actually create a feeling of postworkout euphoria as blood circulates throughout your muscles.

In weight training, intensity is defined as the amount of work performed in a given period of time—in essence, it is a function of how hard you train. Thus, training at 100 percent intensity would mean that you physically could not perform even one more repetition. There are two facets of exercise intensity: the amount of weight used (workload) and the amount of rest in between sets (rest interval). Both can be manipulated to achieve a desired result.

Workload

All too often, women train with weights that are not heavy enough to evoke a satisfactory muscular response. Generally, this is due to the accepted theory that women should train with "light" weights so that they won't bulk up. Unfortunately, this advice has been misconstrued to mean that there should not be muscular discomfort during training when nothing could be further from the truth.

Muscles only respond when subjected to an intense stress. If a muscle is not sufficiently taxed, there is no impetus for muscular development. Consequently, you must use a weight that causes you to struggle on the last few reps of a set. While the weights that you use will be "light" on an absolute basis, they should feel "heavy" by the time you complete your set.

You must learn to withstand the temporary discomfort associated with this type of training. Fortunately, the pain is only transitory, dissipating as soon as you finish your set. Exercise-induced discomfort is largely a psychological function and can be regulated by developing the proper mind-set. By having the appropriate perspective and enduring this short-term anguish, you will reap tremendous rewards from your efforts.

Rest Intervals

In order to enhance a feminine physique, this routine uses limited *rest intervals* of about 30 seconds between sets. A rest interval is the time that elapses from the point at which you finish a set to the moment you start your next set. The shorter the rest interval, the greater the intensity of exercise.

Limiting your rest intervals will help to reduce overall body fat. By training in a more continuous fashion, you give your workout more of an aerobic effect and substantially increase total calories burned. As previously stated, this will significantly improve fat mobilization and help to produce a lean, toned physique.

An additional benefit of limited rest intervals is that they reduce the amount of time needed to work out. Your entire weight-training session will last no more than twenty minutes! Thus, no matter how busy your schedule, you will always have the opportunity to get in a workout.

To maximize the use of the time between sets, this routine employs a technique called selective muscular stretching, which allows you to improve flexibility while increasing your strength. Upon completion of a set, immediately stretch the muscle being trained utilizing the stretching movements discussed below. Try to hold each stretch throughout the entire rest interval and then proceed directly to your next set.

When you stretch, go only to the point where you feel tension in the muscle—not to where you experience unbearable pain. If you stretch too far, your body sends a neural impulse to the over-stretched muscle, causing it to contract. This reflex actually tightens the muscle, creating the opposite effect of what you are trying to accomplish. By stretching slowly, you can ease into a comfortable zone, taking your body to the edge without going over.

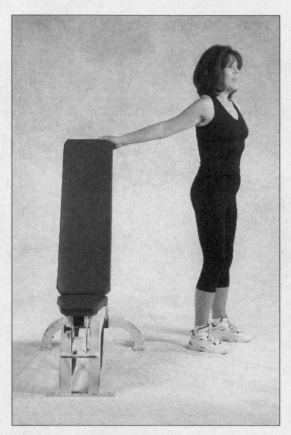

FIGURE 6.1 CHEST STRETCH

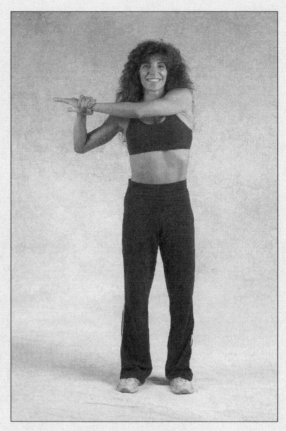

FIGURE 6.2 SHOULDER STRETCH

Chest Stretch: From a standing position, grasp any stationary object (such as an exercise bench) with your right hand. Your arm should be straight and roughly parallel with the ground. Slowly turn your body away from the object, allowing your arm to go as far behind your body as comfortably possible. Hold this position for 15 seconds and repeat this process on the left.

Shoulder Stretch: From a standing position, grasp your right wrist with your left hand. Without turning your body, slowly pull your right arm across your torso as far as comfortably possibly. Hold this position for 15 seconds and repeat the process on the left.

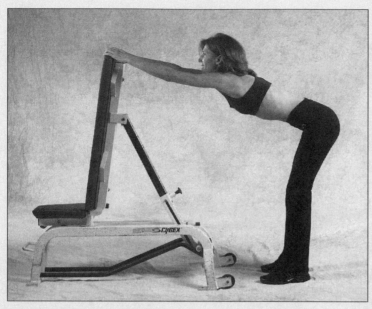

FIGURE 6.3 LAT STRETCH

Lat Stretch: From a standing position, grasp any stationary object (such as an exercise bench) with both hands at chest level. Bend your knees slightly and sit back so that your arms are fully extended and supporting your weight. Shift your weight to the right in order to isolate the right portion of your latissimus dorsi muscle. Hold this position for 15 seconds and then shift your weight to the left.

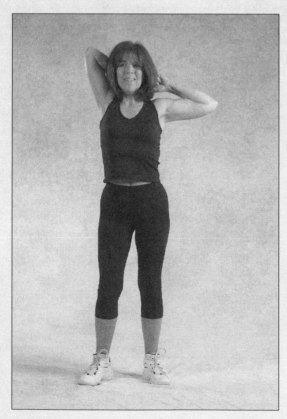

FIGURE 6.4 TRICEPS STRETCH

Triceps Stretch: From a standing position, raise your right arm over your head. Bend your elbow so that your right hand is behind your head. With your left hand, grasp your right wrist or hand and pull it back as far as comfortably possible, allowing your elbow to point toward the ceiling. Hold this position for 15 seconds and repeat this process on the left.

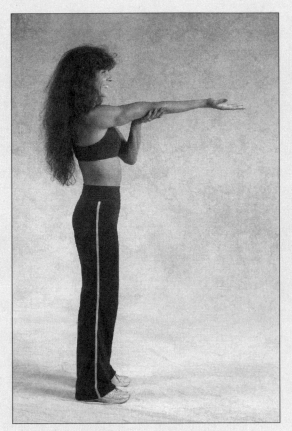

FIGURE 6.5 BICEPS STRETCH

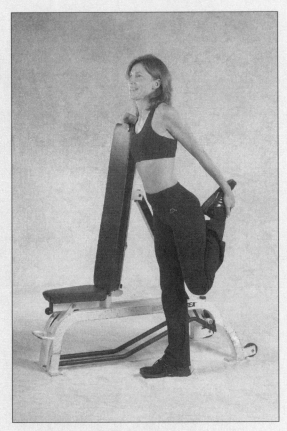

FIGURE 6.6 QUADRICEPS STRETCH

Biceps Stretch: From a standing position, extend your right arm forward with your palm facing up. Place your left palm underneath your right elbow. Slowly straighten your right arm as much as comfortably possible, pressing your elbow down into your left hand. Hold this position for 15 seconds and repeat this process on the left.

Quadriceps Stretch: From a standing position, grasp a stationary object (such as an exercise bench) with your left hand. Bend your right knee, bringing your right foot toward your butt. Grasp your right foot or ankle with your right hand and slowly pull your foot upward as high and as comfortably possible. Hold this position for 15 seconds and repeat this process on the left.

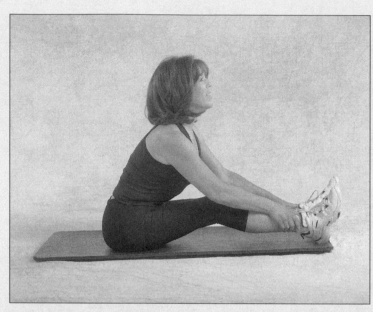

FIGURE 6.7 HAMSTRINGS STRETCH

Hamstrings Stretch: From a seated position, straighten your legs in front of you and slowly bend forward at the waist. Allow your hands to travel downward along the line of your body as far as comfortably possible. At the point where you feel an intense stretch in your hamstrings, grab onto your legs and hold this position for 30 seconds.

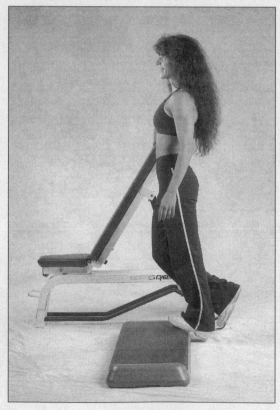

FIGURE 6.8 CALF STRETCH

Calf Stretch: Stand on a raised block of wood or a step platform and grasp a stationary object for balance. Take your left foot off of the block so that you are standing on your right leg. Slowly allow your right heel to travel downward as far as comfortably possible. Hold this position for 15 seconds and repeat the process on the left.

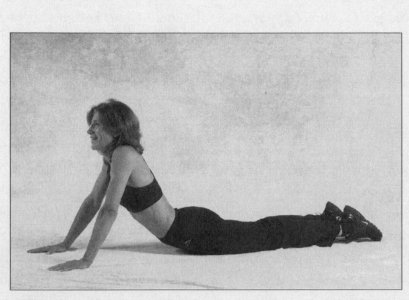

Abdominal Stretch: Lie down on your stomach with your palms on the floor at your sides. Keeping your pelvis pressed to the floor, slowly push your upper body up until your arms are fully straightened. Hold this position for 30 seconds.

FIGURE 6.9 ABDOMINAL STRETCH

Acclimation

While intense training is fundamental to your progress, you must start slowly and deliberately build up your intensity levels. Gradually increasing intensity in a systematic fashion will prevent trauma to your muscle tissue, which can derail your workout regimen and impede your progress. Although you probably are anxious to get results, you must train within your own capabilities. Doing so will ensure a safe and effective workout.

During your first week of training, you should choose weights that do not tax your resources and take as long as needed between sets. The weights utilized should comprise no more than 50 percent of your absolute strength levels so that you can comfortably finish each set without struggling. Moreover, you should allow your heart rate to return to resting levels before beginning your next set. These workouts should not be laborious, and you should not feel depleted after the session.

In the second week, you should attempt to slightly increase the amount of weight used and slightly decrease the amount of rest between sets. Assess how this affects your body and make adjustments based on your physical state. While you should experience a mild degree of soreness for one or two days after each session, you shouldn't be physically debilitated. If your soreness does limit you physically, proceed a little more slowly, using lighter weights. Alternatively, if you aren't sore at all, you probably can increase your intensity a little more. Either way, do not become impatient and always progress at your own pace.

As each succeeding week passes, you should continue to raise your intensity so that you become significantly challenged by the workouts. Within a few months, the weights utilized should tax your strength abilities, making it a struggle to complete your sets. (You should barely be able to get up the last rep). Rest intervals should be limited to about thirty seconds with your heart rate elevated throughout the session.

Frequency

Many women think that they are augmenting muscle tone as they are working out. In fact, training produces quite the opposite effect. Muscle tissue is actually broken down during a workout. Tiny microscopic tears are formed in your muscle and connective tissue during training, which serves to break down muscle. At rest, your body senses that it will again be muscularly stressed in the near future. Thus, your body repairs your muscle tissue (i.e., becomes "toned") in preparation for the next workout. Without rest, your muscles never have a chance to recuperate, making you prone to an overtrained state. Symptoms of overtraining include insomnia, fatigue, decreased motivation to exercise, flu-like symptoms, depression, and increased frequency of injuries. If overtraining occurs, you will cease to make further gains and can even regress in your training efforts.

Since the Look Great at Any Age program is intense, adequate recuperation is essential in order to repair muscle tissue and avoid overtraining. Accordingly, you should perform the routine on three nonconsecutive days per week (i.e., Workout One from chapter 7 on Monday, Workout Two from chapter 8 on Wednesday, and Workout Three from chapter 9 on Friday or Workout One on Tuesday, Workout Two on Thursday, and Workout Three on Saturday, etc.). This allows at least forty-eight hours for your neuromuscular system to regenerate from the previous workout.

Good results can even be achieved with only two days a week of training—especially if you have been completely sedentary for long periods of time. If you decide to employ a twice-weekly schedule, it's best to space out sessions a little more, allowing seventy-two hours of rest between workouts. Hence a Monday/Thursday, Tuesday/Fri, etc., schedule is ideal.

Finally, it is important to listen to your body and make adjustments in your routine based on how you feel. If you are run-down, do not hesitate to take an extra day off. As long as you are disciplined, an extra day or two of rest will not set back your training endeavors, and can often help to rejuvenate your strength and enthusiasm. When in doubt, it is better to train a little less than to overtrain.

CHAPTER 7

Workout One

Fifty-six-year-old Barbara Kaufman, the fitness model for this chapter, never stops running. As the director of a nursery school, she supervises a staff of fifteen people that looks after 135 preschoolers. As if that isn't exhausting enough, she then goes over to her second job working as a counselor with developmentally disabled children.

For Barbara, exercise is a salvation. She first started working out when she was in her late twenties. It was the height of the aerobic craze and she joined the ranks of the many women who were getting aerobicized. But while she saw some positive changes in her body, aerobics simply didn't produce the toned physique that she desired. That's when she decided to hit the weights.

Barbara gets in her workouts whenever she can. Sometimes she trains first thing in the morning, other times immediately after work. After a grueling day, this can be a chore. But Barbara doesn't give in. She forces herself to work out, thinking about how good she'll feel after the session.

In addition to looking and feeling better, Barbara credits exercise with her boundless energy. Her husband calls her the "Energizer Bunny," and most would agree. Not only does the extra energy help her through her busy schedule, but she's also able to keep up with her three children and two grandchildren!

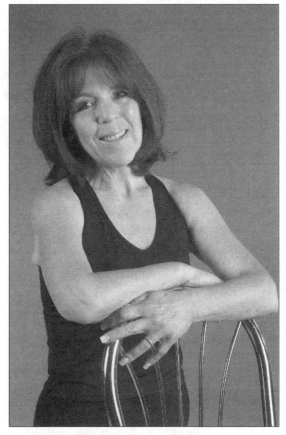

BARBARA KAUFMAN

FLAT DUMBBELL PRESS

Target muscles: *Chest*

Secondary muscles used: *Frontal shoulders and triceps*

Start: Lie faceup on a flat bench, planting your feet firmly on the floor. Grasp two dumbbells and, with your palms facing away from your body, bring them to shoulder level so that they rest just above your armpits.

Movement: Simultaneously press both dumbbells directly over your chest, moving them in toward each other on the ascent. At the finish of the movement, the sides of the dumbbells (next to your thumbs) should gently touch. Feel a contraction in your chest muscles at the top of the movement and then slowly reverse direction, lowering the dumbbells along the same path back to the start position.

Tips:

1. *Don't press out in an arc on the ascent.* You should avoid allowing the weights to move out— creating a "circular" movement. The rotator cuff muscles are unduly stressed from this movement and the shoulder joint is placed in a compromising position. Rather, press the dumbbells in while you are raising the weights, as if you are making a "triangle" with your arms. This will ensure that your chest muscles receive maximal stimulus and allow you to get a better contraction during the lift.

2. *Keep your butt on the bench at all times.* As the set becomes more difficult, a woman often will lift her butt into the air to gain additional leverage. However, this only serves to diminish the involvement of the chest muscles and can cause injury to the lower back. Thus, it is imperative to make sure your butt is pressed into the bench as you are lifting, keeping your body position stable.

3. *Keep your elbows out and back throughout the movement.* When the elbows are kept in close to the body, there is significant activation of the triceps at the expense of the chest muscles. Since it is important to minimize triceps involvement, your elbows should stay virtually perpendicular to your torso during performance.

4. *Don't stretch down too far.* If you overstretch at the bottom of the movement, severe pressure is placed on the upper torso and injury can occur. Accordingly, you should bring your arms down only to a point where you feel a comfortable stretch in your chest muscles without any pain to this area.

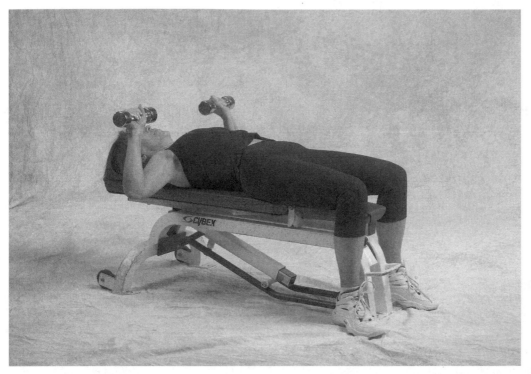

FIGURE 7.1 FLAT DUMBBELL PRESS

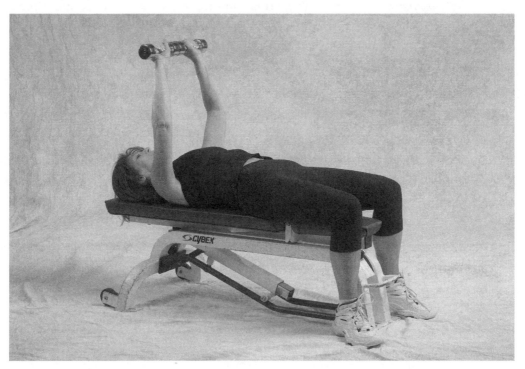

FIGURE 7.2 FLAT DUMBBELL PRESS

WORKOUT ONE

ONE-ARM DUMBBELL ROW

Target muscles: *Back*

Secondary muscles used: *Rear shoulders, biceps, and forearms*

Start: Placing your left hand and left knee on a flat bench, keep your right foot planted firmly on the floor. Your torso should be parallel with the floor throughout the entire movement. Grasp a dumbbell in your right hand and, with your palm facing the side of your body, let it hang down to the floor.

Movement: Keeping your elbow close to your body, pull the dumbbell upward and back until it touches your hip. Feel a contraction in the muscles of your upper back and slowly reverse direction, lowering the dumbbell along the same path back to the start position. After you have finished the desired number of repetitions, invert the process and perform an equal number of reps with your left arm.

Tips:

   1. *Don't round your back while lifting.* It is common for a woman to round her back during performance, especially toward the end of a set. This reduces the ability to contract the upper back muscles and places a great deal of stress on the lower back. To ensure that your body remains parallel to the floor, it is beneficial to keep your straight leg back at an angle. This gives you a greater center of balance and provides less ability to raise your torso.

   2. *Don't allow your arm to gravitate away from your body.* When you swing your arm outward to pull up the weight, the shoulders and arms become increasingly active in the move. The joints and connective tissue are excessively stressed, heightening injury to this area. In order to keep tension in the muscles of the upper back, your elbow must remain close to your torso, resulting in a straight-line upward pull.

   3. *Make sure you achieve a full stretch at the bottom of the movement.* This is one of the few exercises during which you can lock out your elbow without ill effect. Doing so will allow the muscles of the upper back to uncoil fully, promoting better development. In order to accentuate a stretch to this area, let the weight drift slightly forward on the descent.

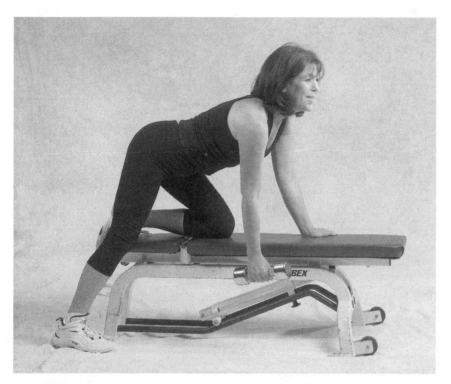

FIGURE 7.3 ONE-ARM DUMBBELL ROW

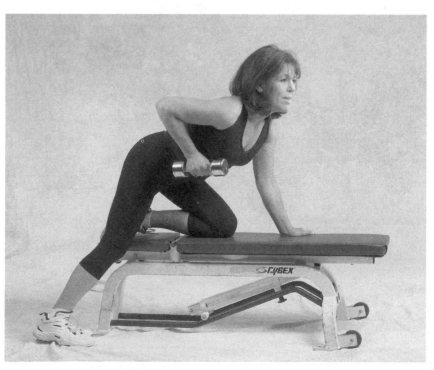

FIGURE 7.4 ONE-ARM DUMBBELL ROW

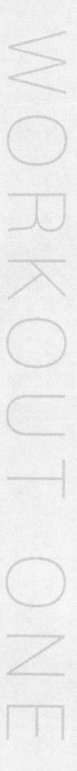

WORKOUT ONE

WORKOUT ONE

SEATED DUMBBELL OVERHEAD PRESS

Target muscles: *Shoulders*

Secondary muscles used: *Upper back and triceps*

Start: Sit upright on the edge of a flat bench with your feet planted firmly on the floor. Grasp one dumbbell in each hand and, with your palms facing away from your body, bring them to shoulder level so that they rest just above the outer region of your shoulders.

Movement: Simultaneously press both dumbbells directly over your head, moving them in toward each other on the ascent. At the finish of the movement, the sides of the dumbbells (next to your thumbs) should gently touch. Feel a contraction in your shoulder muscles at the top of the movement and then slowly reverse direction, lowering the dumbbells along the same path back to the start position.

Tips:

1. *Don't allow the weights to move out in an arc as you are pressing.* As in the flat dumbbell press, raising the weights in a circular motion places undue stress on the shoulder joint, subjecting it to potential injury. Thus, you must press the dumbbells in as you are raising the weights, keeping the movement as compact as possible.

2. *Make sure you press straight up during the lift.* A frequent mistake made is lifting the weights in either a forward or backward direction, which puts the shoulder joint in a compromising position. Watching your performance in a mirror can often throw off your sense of distance, compounding this inclination. You must lift the weights directly overhead, creating a straight line with the floor. If the mirror hinders your performance ability, close your eyes and visualize the movement until it becomes second nature.

3. *Keep your shoulders relaxed throughout the move.* It is common to tense up during this exercise, causing stiffness in the neck and trapezius. To alleviate this tendency, it is important to stay loose while lifting. It can be helpful to take several deep breaths before beginning the movement, and if you find yourself tensing during the lift, stop training immediately.

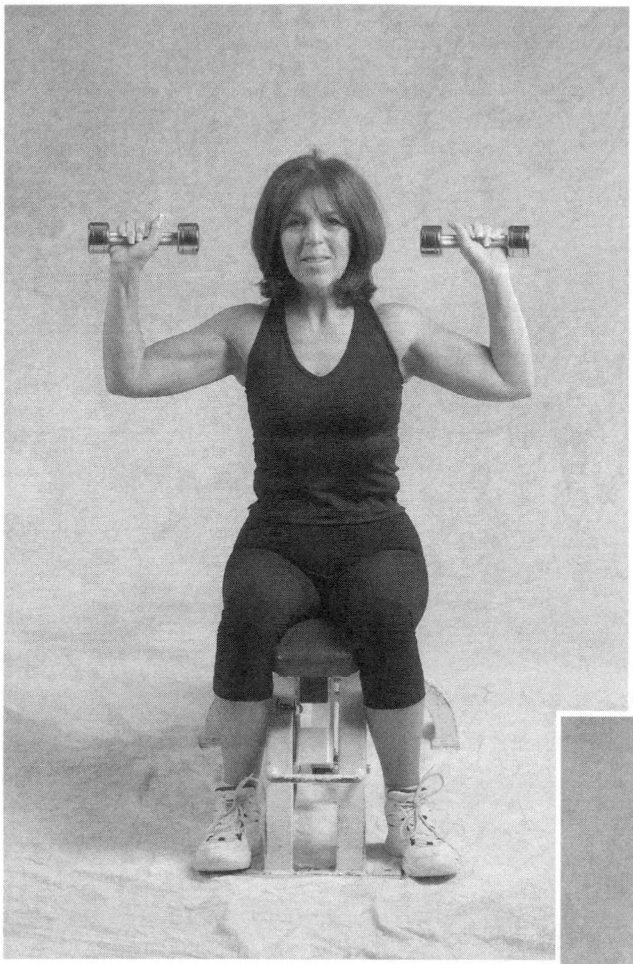

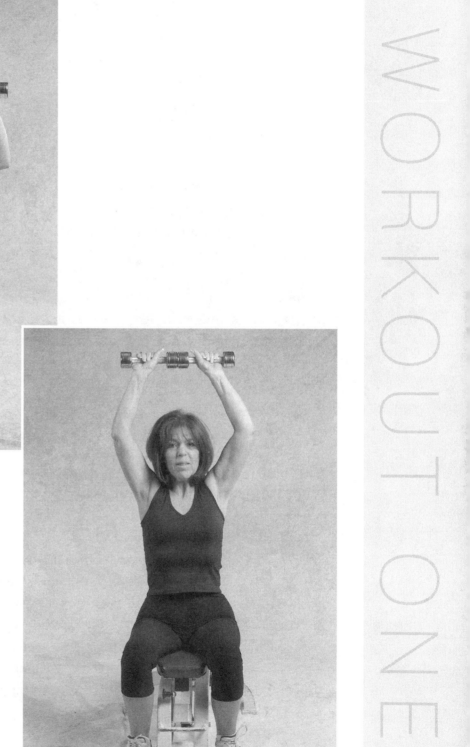

FIGURE 7.5 SEATED DUMBBELL OVERHEAD PRESS

FIGURE 7.6 SEATED DUMBBELL OVERHEAD PRESS

WORKOUT ONE

WORKOUT-ONE

SEATED DUMBBELL CURL

Target muscles: *Biceps*

Secondary muscles used: *Forearms*

Start: Sit upright on the edge of a flat bench with your feet planted firmly on the floor. Grasp a dumbbell in each hand and, with your palms facing away from your body, let them rest at your sides. Press your upper arms against your torso and maintain this position throughout the movement.

Movement: Simultaneously raise the dumbbells forward and up, continuing until your hands stop just short of your shoulders. Feel a contraction in your biceps at the top of the movement and then slowly reverse direction, lowering the weight along the same path back to the start position.

Tips:

1. *Keep your wrists taut during the lift.* Since women typically have weak wrists, maintaining stability in this area often becomes problematic. Consequently, during biceps movements, it is common to roll the wrists during performance. This removes stress from the biceps and transfers it to the muscles of the forearms. In order to counteract this effect, you must avoid letting your wrists bend downward, locking them in a fixed position throughout the move.

2. *Don't allow your elbows to rise up during performance.* Because the biceps are such a small muscle complex, they require isolation for proper development. However, when the upper arms extend forward, the shoulders become the primary muscle movers, significantly reducing biceps stimulus. It is therefore important to keep your elbows pointed down and your upper arm perpendicular to the floor. This will assure that the biceps perform the majority of the work.

3. *Never lean back while lifting.* In order to obtain additional leverage, it is common to swing the body backward during the movement. However, cheating the weight up in this fashion does little to enhance biceps development and can be injurious to the lower back. Hence, your body must remain erect as you curl the weight. If you have an adjustable bench, set it in an upright position. This will prevent your body from swaying and provide adequate back support during the move.

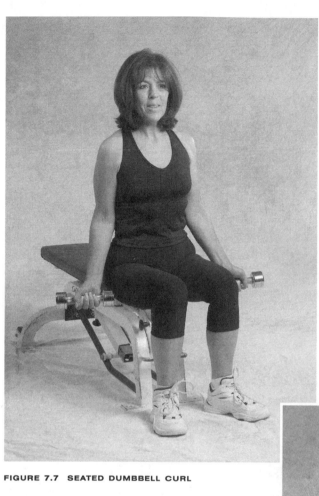

FIGURE 7.7 SEATED DUMBBELL CURL

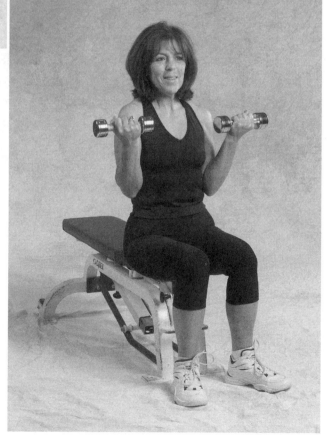

FIGURE 7.8 SEATED DUMBBELL CURL

WORKOUT ONE

TRICEPS KICKBACK

Target muscles: *Triceps*

Secondary muscles used: *None*

Start: While standing, bend at the waist and tilt your body forward so that your torso is roughly parallel with the floor. Your knees should be slightly bent. Grasp a dumbbell in each hand and, with your palms facing your body, bring your upper arms in line with your torso and bend your elbows so that your forearms are approximately perpendicular to the floor. Press your upper arms against your body and maintain this position throughout the movement.

Movement: Simultaneously raise the dumbbells until your forearms are completely straightened and parallel with the ground. Feel a contraction in your triceps at the top of the movement and then slowly reverse direction, lowering the weights along the same path back to the start position.

Tips:

1. *Don't swing your upper arm.* All too frequently, a woman will use her shoulder in the performance of the movement, swinging her arm as she lifts the weight. Unfortunately, the triceps are a relatively small muscle complex and receive very little stimulus from this action. The only part of your body that should move is your forearm, keeping the upper arm perfectly still at all times.

2. *Keep your upper arms parallel with the floor throughout the lift.* As your arms become fatigued, it is common to let them progressively drift downward, decreasing the effect of the exercise. By keeping your arms parallel, you will ensure that your muscles work against gravity for maximum resistance. If you can't maintain this position, you're probably using too much weight and should adjust your workload accordingly.

3. *Keep your wrists taut, especially at the top of the movement.* In the quest to fully contract the triceps, there is a tendency for a woman to inadvertently flick her wrists as she straightens her arms. Not only does this hamper performance, but it also puts a strain on the wrists themselves. Thus, you should lock your wrists into a fixed position throughout the move, keeping them on the same plane as the rest of your arms.

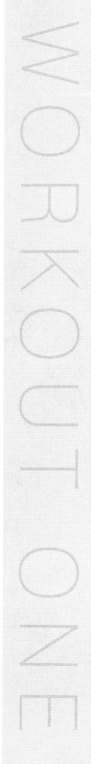

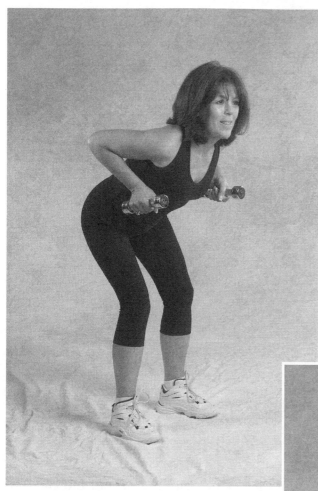

FIGURE 7.9 TRICEPS KICKBACK

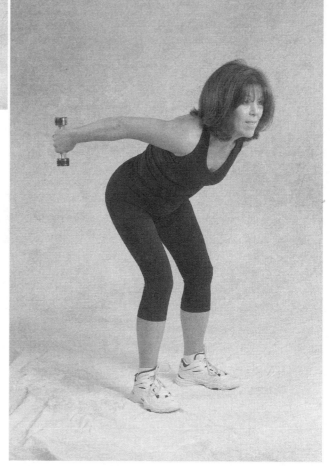

FIGURE 7.10 TRICEPS KICKBACK

DUMBBELL LUNGE

Target muscles: *Quadriceps*

Secondary muscles used: *Hamstrings and glutes*

Start: Stand upright with a shoulder-width stance and your left foot approximately three feet in front of you. Raise your right heel off the floor, point your toes forward, and maintain a slight bend to both knees. Grasp a dumbbell in each hand and, with palms facing in toward the sides of your body, allow them to hang at your sides.

Movement: Bend your left knee, allowing your right knee to descend downward toward the floor. Just before your right knee touches the floor, feel a contraction in the muscles of the front of this leg and then slowly reverse direction, rising up along the same path back to start position. After you have finished the desired number of repetitions, invert the process and perform an equal number of reps with the other leg.

Tips:

1. *Never allow your front knee to pass over the plane of your toe.* Do not push your front knee forward as you lower your rear leg. This overextends the front knee, placing a great deal of pressure on the joint. Rather, you must drop your rear leg straight down, keeping your front shin perpendicular throughout the move.

2. *Keep your rear heel elevated throughout the movement.* When the heel of your rear leg is flat, much of the tension is removed from the quadriceps. Since continuous tension is imperative to maximizing results, this reduces the effectiveness of the exercise. It is better to maintain a raised heel at all times, keeping all your weight on your toes. If you cannot hold this position for a full set, attempt to do it for several reps at a time, working up to your target rep range.

3. *Don't lean forward during the lift.* When performing this move, it is often difficult to maintain balance. In order to rectify this problem, you should keep your shoulders back and chin up. Look straight ahead or even up in the air—not down at the ground. This will prevent you from falling forward and will help you keep your balance at all times.

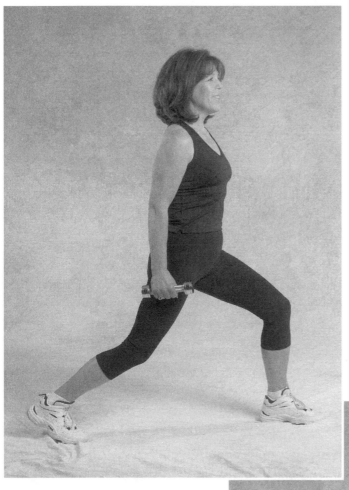

FIGURE 7.11 DUMBBELL LUNGE

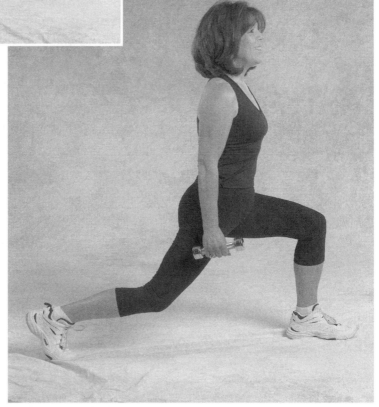

FIGURE 7.12 DUMBBELL LUNGE

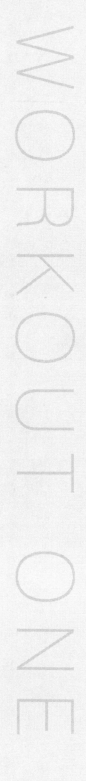

WORKOUT ONE

STIFF-LEGGED DEADLIFT

Target muscles: *Hamstrings, glutes*

Secondary muscles used: *Lower back*

Start: Standing upright, maintain a shoulder-width stance with your knees straightened. Hold a dumbbell in both hands in front of your torso with your palms facing the front of your body.

Movement: Bend your torso forward at the hips and allow the dumbbells to travel downward along the line of your body. Continue this descent until you feel a distinct stretch in the backs of your legs. Slowly reverse direction and contract your glutes as you rise up along the same path back to the start position.

Tips:

1. *Don't pull up with your arms or shrug your shoulders during the movement.* If you allow your upper body to assist in the performance of the move, you will reduce stress to the target muscles of the lower body. For proper execution, your upper body should remain lifeless, like a rag doll. Think of your arms only as hooks that hold the weights during the lift with all movement generating from your hips.

2. *Keep the weights close to your body at all times.* When the weights are allowed to drift away from the body, the lower back becomes increasingly involved in the movement. Ultimately, this area is subjected to excessive stress and injury can occur. In order to keep the focus on your butt and hamstrings, never let the weights travel more than a few inches from your body.

3. *Don't fully straighten your body at the start position.* By bringing the body into an erect position, stress is taken off the glutes and transferred to the lower back. To reverse this effect, you should stop just short of perpendicular, maintaining a slight forward lean to your body.

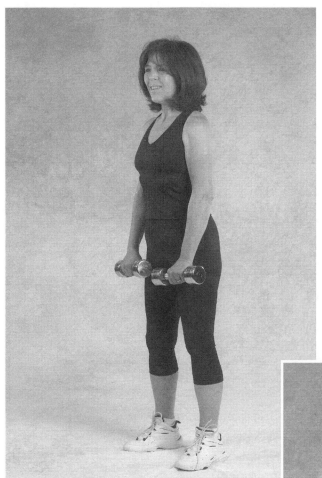

FIGURE 7.13 STIFF-LEGGED DEADLIFT

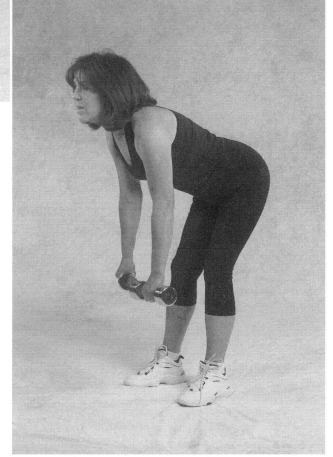

FIGURE 7.14 STIFF-LEGGED DEADLIFT

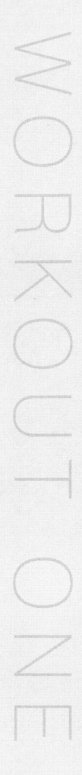

STANDING HEEL RAISE

Target muscles: *Calves*

Secondary muscles used: *None*

Start: Begin by standing upright with your feet about shoulder-width apart and hold a dumbbell in your right hand.

Movement: Simultaneously raise your heels as high as possible, transferring your weight to the balls of your feet. Feel a contraction in your calf muscles and then slowly reverse direction, descending along the same path back to the start position.

Tips:

1. *Don't lean forward during the move.* There is a tendency to tilt to the front as the heels are elevated. This can cause you to lose balance and fall forward. Therefore, keep your body completely erect as you ascend, centering your weight so that balance is maintained.

2. *Place your hands against a stationary object for extra support.* If you have difficulty maintaining your equilibrium, you should lightly place your fingers against a wall or a raised bench as you perform the move. After a short period of time, your balance will improve and you will be able to execute the lift without support.

3. *Perform the move on stairs for increased resistance.* When you can easily perform the target number of repetitions, it is beneficial to execute the move on the bottom step of a staircase. By placing your feet on the edge of the step, you can allow your heels to stretch down, significantly increasing your range of motion. In this version, make sure to hold on to the banister for support.

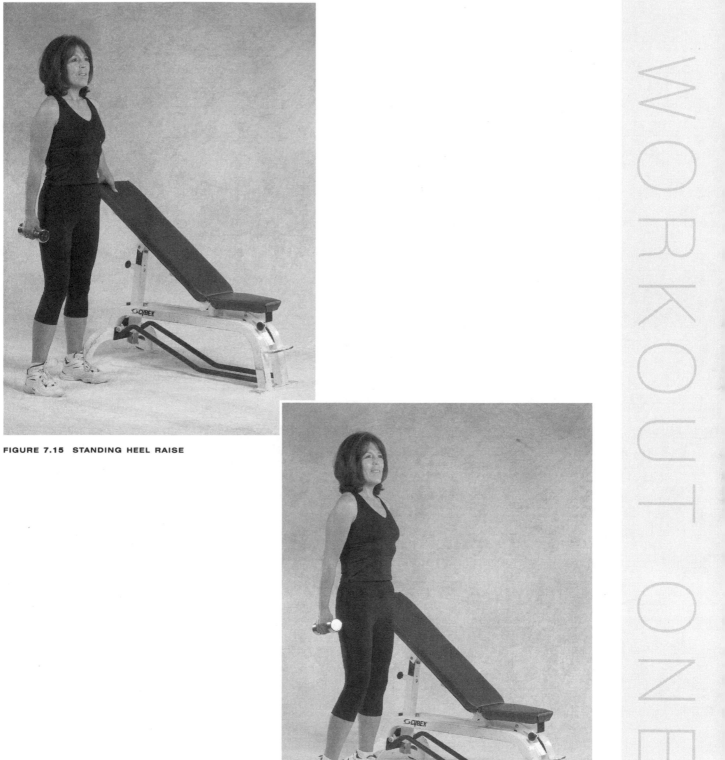

FIGURE 7.15 STANDING HEEL RAISE

FIGURE 7.16 STANDING HEEL RAISE

WORKOUT ONE

CRUNCH

Target muscles: *Abdominals*

Secondary muscles used: *None*

Start: Begin by lying faceup on the floor with your knees bent. Your hands should be folded across your chest. You can also try resting your calves on top of a flat bench so that your thighs are perpendicular to the floor.

Movement: Slowly raise your shoulders up and forward toward your chest, shortening the distance of your trunk. Feel a contraction in your abdominal muscles and then slowly reverse direction, rising up along the same path back to the start position.

Tips:

1. *Don't place your hands behind your head.* Even many fitness professionals wrongly advise supporting your head with your hands. Unfortunately, doing so often causes a woman to reflexively pull up from the head, rather than the abs, and can lead to a strain or pull of the neck muscles. It is better to keep your hands on your chest and tuck your chin down as you raise your body. This will alleviate pressure on the neck and force the abs to perform the lift.

2. *Your lower back must stay on the ground at all times.* Unlike the sit-up, crunches are a very compact move during which the lower back should not rise up during performance. This helps to remove involvement of the hip-flexor muscles and therefore keeps continuous tension on the abs. To perform the lift correctly, you must press your lower back into the floor and pull up only from the shoulders.

3. *When it becomes easy to perform the given number of reps, utilize a weight for added resistance.* There is little utility in performing more than twenty reps of an exercise. This merely impedes concentration and makes the move a purely aerobic endeavor. Thus, when you develop considerable abdominal strength, it is beneficial to hold a dumbbell across your chest as you perform the move.

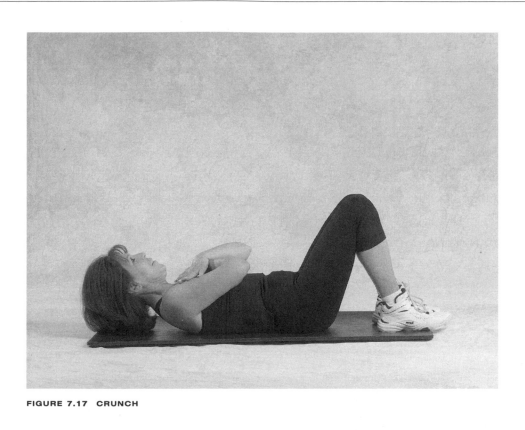

FIGURE 7.17 CRUNCH

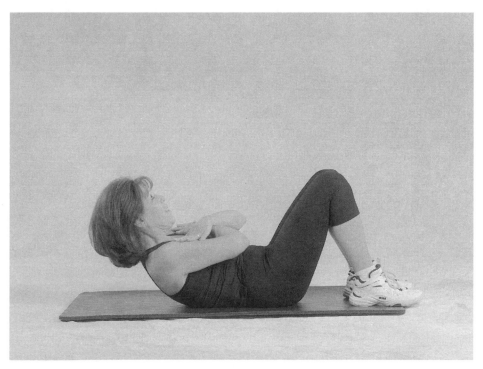

FIGURE 7.18 CRUNCH

WORKOUT ONE

SUMMARY: WORKOUT ONE

Table 7.1 summarizes the specifics of Workout One. Since everyone has different initial strength and fitness levels, you should use the suggested starting weights only as a guide and adjust them according to your individual strength levels. If you have never trained before and do not have someone who will supervise your workout and demonstrate proper exercise form, it can be beneficial to begin simply by learning the performance of each exercise without any weights. Do this as long as it takes to understand each movement.

Table 7.1

WORKOUT ONE					
MUSCLE GROUP	**EXERCISE**	**REPS**	**SETS**	**REST INTERVAL**	**STARTING WEIGHT**
CHEST	Flat Dumbbell Press	15 to 20	1	30 Seconds	5
UPPER BACK	One-Arm Dumbbell Row	15 to 20	1	30 Seconds	8
SHOULDERS	Overhead Dumbbell Press	15 to 20	1	30 Seconds	5
BICEPS	Seated Dumbbell Curl	15 to 20	1	30 Seconds	5
TRICEPS	Triceps Kickbacks	15 to 20	1	30 Seconds	3
QUADRICEPS	Lunge	15 to 20	1	30 Seconds	3
HAMS/GLUTES	Stiff-Legged Deadlift	15 to 20	1	30 Seconds	8
CALVES	Heel Raise	15 to 20	1	30 Seconds	5
ABDOMINALS	Crunch	15 to 20	1	30 Seconds	No Weight

WORKOUT ONE

CHAPTER 8

Workout Two

Annette Saleski, the fitness model for this chapter, is a true inspiration. Always active in her teens (she was a cheerleader), the effects of partying after high school left her twenty pounds overweight and dissatisfied with her physique. What's more, as a self-proclaimed hyperactive person, she started having frequent panic attacks. By the time she turned twenty-five, she decided to tackle her problems through exercise.

Today, at forty-two, Annette equates fitness with brushing her teeth: It's something she simply has to do. Feeling that her energy levels are highest in the morning, she likes to work out as soon as she gets up; by 6 A.M., she's already hitting the weights. After that, it's off to her job as the administrator of a busy construction company.

Annette exemplifies the benefits of leading a fitness lifestyle. She is lean and defined, with a strong, shapely physique. The panic attacks are gone, and her mental state is significantly improved. And, best of all, no one can believe that she's in her forties!

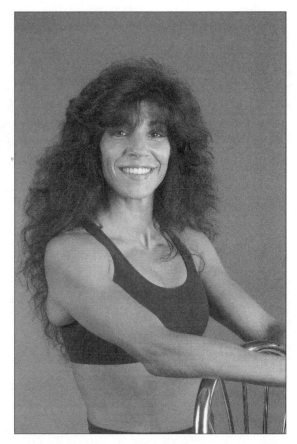

ANNETTE SALESKI

INCLINE DUMBBELL FLYE

Target muscles: *Chest*

Secondary muscles used: *Frontal shoulders and triceps*

Start: Lie faceup on an incline with your feet planted firmly on the floor. Grasp two dumbbells and bring them out to your sides, maintaining a slight bend to your elbows throughout the move. Your palms should be facing in and toward the ceiling, and your upper arms should be roughly parallel with the level of the bench.

Movement: Slowly raise the weights upward in a semicircular motion, as if you were hugging a large tree. Gently touch the weights together at the top of the move and, after feeling a contraction in your chest muscles, slowly return the weights along the same path back to the start position.

Tips:

   1. *Set the bench at a moderate incline.* The degree of bench incline has a direct bearing on which muscles are activated during training. If the incline is too steep, an inordinate amount of work is transferred to the shoulder muscles (which are not the target muscles in this exercise). For maximum stimulation of the target muscles of the chest, keep the incline set at about 30 to 35 degrees.

   2. *Keep your arms fixed throughout the move.* One of the most common mistakes made during performance of the flye is to flex and extend the arms. This effectively turns the exercise into a pressing movement, thereby negating isolation-oriented benefits. For best results, movement should take place only at the shoulder joint; the arms must remain rigid at all times.

   3. *Don't allow your butt to rise up during chest training.* Lifting your butt off the bench may help to improve leverage, but it also reduces the amount of stress applied to the pectoral muscles. What's more, the lower back is placed in a precarious position, heightening the potential for injury. To maximize performance, your butt should remain pressed to the bench at all times. Use only the target muscles to lift the weights and avoid any extraneous movement of the lower body or torso.

   4. *Don't overstretch at the start position.* If you allow your arms to stretch down too far at the bottom of the movement, severe pressure is placed on the shoulder joint and injury can occur. You should bring your arms down only to a point where you feel a comfortable stretch in the chest muscles without any pain to this area—generally no lower than a point where your upper arms are parallel with the floor.

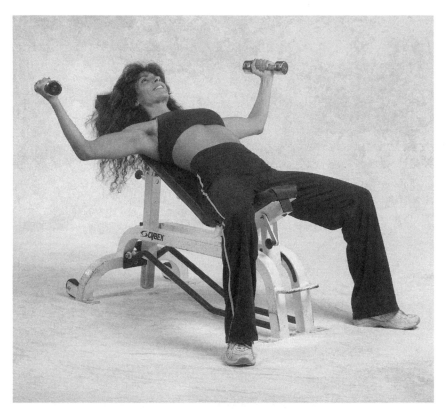

FIGURE 8.1 INCLINE DUMBBELL FLYE

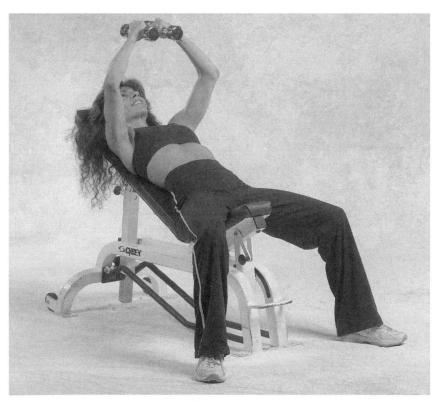

FIGURE 8.2 INCLINE DUMBBELL FLYE

WORKOUT TWO

DUMBBELL PULLOVER

Target muscles: *Back*

Secondary muscles used: *Lower chest, triceps*

Start: Lie back on a flat bench. Grasp a dumbbell with both hands and bring it to a position directly over your face.

Movement: Keeping your arms slightly bent, slowly lower the dumbbell behind your head as far as comfortably possible, feeling a complete stretch in your lats. Reverse direction and return the dumbbell back to the start position, squeezing your lats on the ascent.

Tips:

1. *Don't put your feet up on the bench.* While it may be more comfortable to keep your feet on the bench when performing pullovers, it reduces the natural lumbar curvature of the spine and increases pressure on the lower back. Additionally, stability while lifting is impaired, increasing your risk of losing balance, especially when struggling to complete the last few reps of a set. The safest bet is to keep your feet planted firmly on the floor. Make sure they remain grounded throughout the entire set.

2. *Don't stretch down too far.* The shoulder socket is very fragile; any extreme stretch can place an inordinate amount of pressure on the supporting muscles and connective tissue, potentially causing a serious injury. You should bring your arms down only to a point where you feel a comfortable stretch. For most, it is not necessary to lower the weight below a position parallel to the floor.

3. *Don't lock out your arms.* On the concentric (positive) portion of the rep, there is a tendency to lift the weight by extending the elbow. This, however, only serves to unduly activate the triceps and take stress away from the target muscles of the back. Rather, focus on pulling the weight up from the shoulder girdle, keeping your arms stable at all times.

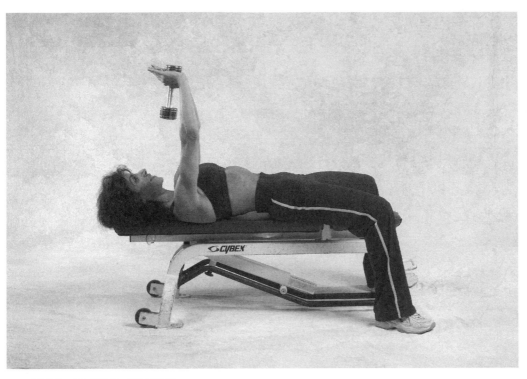

FIGURE 8.3 DUMBBELL PULLOVER

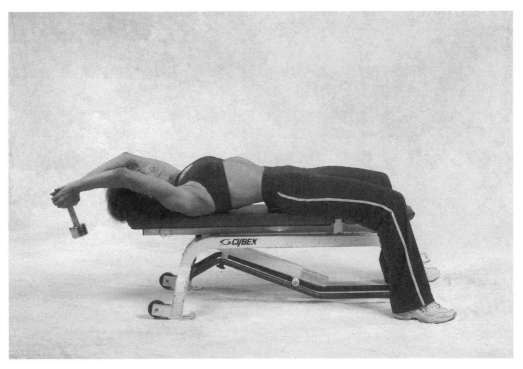

FIGURE 8.4 DUMBBELL PULLOVER

WORKOUT TWO

ARNOLD PRESS

Target muscles: *Shoulders*

Secondary muscles used: *Triceps*

Start: Sit at the edge of a flat bench. Grasp two dumbbells and bring the weights to shoulder level with your palms facing toward your body (as if you had just finished a dumbbell curl).

Movement: Press the dumbbells directly upward, simultaneously rotating your hands so that your palms face forward during the last portion of the movement. Touch the weights together over your head and then slowly return them along the same arc, rotating your hands back to the start position.

Tips:

1. *Perform the movement in a smooth fashion.* Because of the coordination involved, this is a tricky exercise. All too often, people perform the maneuver robotically, as if it were several distinct movements strewn together. Rather, the motion should be smooth—not mechanical. Start turning the weights from the beginning so that, by the time you are midway through the move, your palms face each other; you don't want to wait until the finish of the move to initiate rotation.

2. *Make sure you press straight up during the lift.* Lifting the weights in either a forward or backward direction puts the shoulder joint in a compromising position. Watching your performance in a mirror can often throw off your sense of distance, compounding this inclination. Rather, you must lift the weights directly overhead, creating a straight line with the floor. If the mirror hinders your performance ability, close your eyes and visualize the movement until it becomes second nature.

3. *Keep your shoulders relaxed throughout the move.* It is common to tense up during this exercise, causing stiffness in the neck and trapezius. To alleviate this tendency, it is important to stay loose while lifting. It can be helpful to take several deep breaths before beginning the movement, and if you find yourself tensing during the lift, stop training immediately.

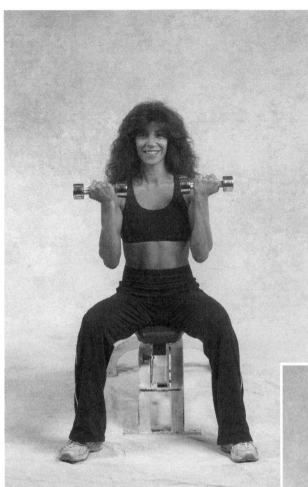

FIGURE 8.5 ARNOLD PRESS

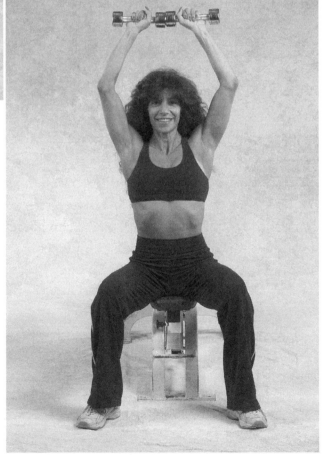

FIGURE 8.6 ARNOLD PRESS

INCLINE DUMBBELL CURL

Target muscles: *Biceps*

Secondary muscles used: *Forearms*

Start: Lie back on an incline bench. Grasp two dumbbells and allow the weights to hang by your hips with your palms facing forward.

Movement: Keeping your upper arms stable, slowly curl the dumbbells upward toward your shoulders. Make sure your elbows stay back throughout the movement. Contract your biceps, then slowly return the weights to the start position.

Tips:

1. *Don't lock your elbows.* All too often, people completely straighten their arms at the start of this move. Locking your elbows not only takes stress away from the target muscle but it also makes the joint susceptible to injury. You should always maintain a slight elbow bend when lowering the weight.

2. *Stay back on the bench.* In an order to make the move easier, there is a tendency to lift the torso off the bench so that it is perpendicular to the floor. This, however, reduces the stretch on the biceps and therefore diminishes muscular force. To maintain maximal stress on your biceps, make sure that your upper back remains pressed to the bench throughout the move, keeping your lower lumbar region in slight hyperextension (normal lumbar curvature).

3. *Don't allow your upper arms to move forward.* Flexing the shoulder joint during this exercise brings ancillary muscles into play, thereby hindering the development of the biceps. To keep stress solely on the biceps, force your upper arms backward and keep them pressed into your sides throughout the move.

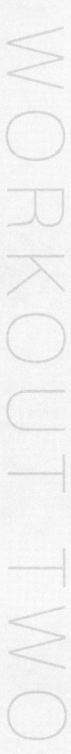

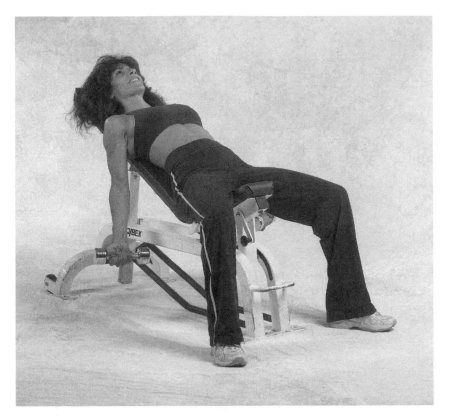

FIGURE 8.7 INCLINE DUMBBELL CURL

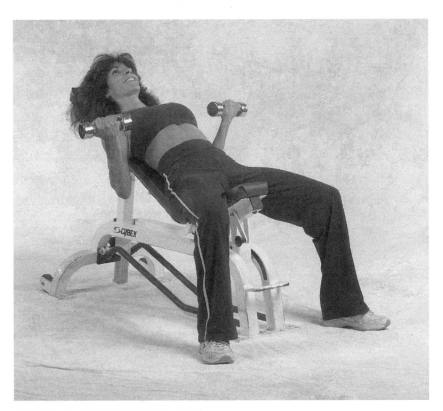

FIGURE 8.8 INCLINE DUMBBELL CURL

WORKOUT TWO

TWO-ARM OVERHEAD DUMBBELL EXTENSION

Target muscles: *Triceps*

Secondary muscles used: *None*

Start: Grasp the stem of a dumbbell with both hands. Bend your elbows and allow the weight to hang down behind your head as far as comfortably possible.

Movement: Slowly straighten your arms, keeping your elbows back and pointed toward the ceiling throughout the move. Contract your triceps and then slowly lower the weight along the same path back to the start position.

Tips:

   1. *Keep your arms in.* There is a tendency to turn your arms outward during performance of this move. While this makes this exercise easier, it also reduces activation of the triceps. Hence, make sure that your upper arms remain pressed into your ears at all times.

   2. *Don't lean backward.* During the eccentric (negative) portion of the rep, the heaviness of the weight can pull your body backward. This can place undue stress on the lumbar region and potentially cause injury. Make sure to stay upright and keep your lower back tight throughout the move.

   3. *Keep your elbows pointed toward the ceiling.* Allowing your upper arms to come forward during performance causes the lats and chest muscles to become excessively activated in the exercise, taking stress away from the target muscles of the triceps. It also can place excessive stress on the elbow joint. For optimal effectiveness, your elbows should remain vertical and pointed toward the ceiling as you lift the weight.

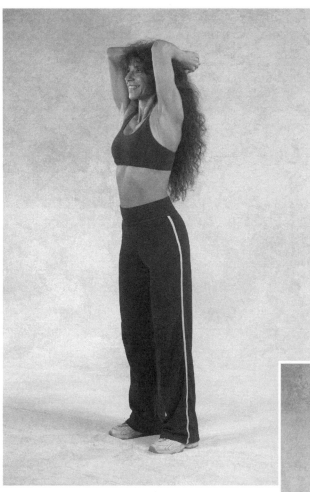

FIGURE 8.9 TWO-ARM OVERHEAD
DUMBBELL EXTENSION

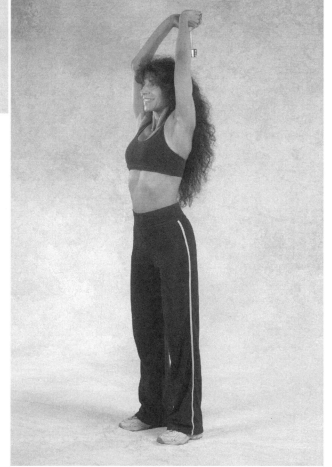

FIGURE 8.10 TWO-ARM OVERHEAD DUMBBELL EXTENSION

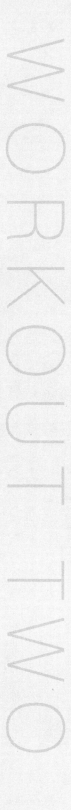

WORKOUT TWO

DUMBBELL SQUAT

Target muscles: *Quadriceps*

Secondary muscles used: *Hamstrings and glutes*

Start: Assume a shoulder-width stance with your toes pointed slightly outward. Grasp two dumbbells and allow them to hang at your sides.

Movement: Slowly lower your body until your thighs are parallel with the floor. Your lower back should be slightly arched and your heels should stay in contact with the floor at all times. When you reach a "seated" position, reverse direction by straightening your legs and return to the start position.

Tips:

1. *Keep your toes pointed slightly outward.* In an effort to stress different parts of the quadriceps, people often experiment with a variety of foot positions. However, since your feet are planted on the floor during the squat, this places undue torque on the knee joint. Instead, point your toes slightly outward at about a 15-degree angle. This allows your patellar tendon to travel in a direct line of pull across the knee joint, preventing excessive stress to the connective tissue.

2. *Never allow your knees to pass over the plane of your toes.* Pushing your knees forward as you lower your torso overextends the knee, placing a great deal of pressure on the joint. Rather, sit back into the move, dropping your butt straight down on the descent.

3. *Keep your chin up.* People tend to lower their heads reflexively as they descend into the squat. This, however, pulls your shoulders downward, causing your back to become rounded (which risks injury to the lumbar region). Hence, make sure that you look straight ahead or even up to the ceiling during the lift.

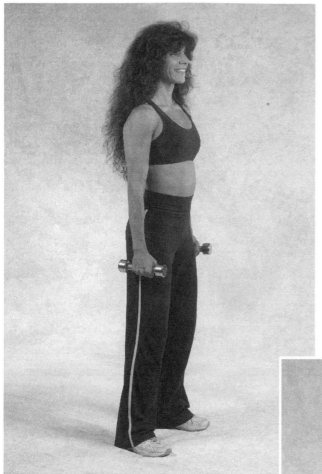

FIGURE 8.11 DUMBBELL SQUAT

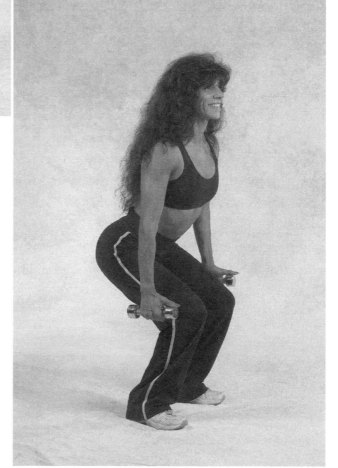

FIGURE 8.12 DUMBBELL SQUAT

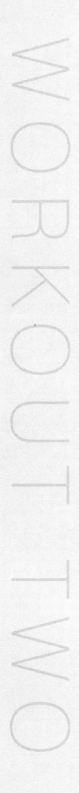

WORKOUT TWO

FLOOR KICK

Target muscles: *Hamstrings, glutes*

Secondary muscles used: *None*

Start: Get into an "all-fours" position, placing your palms on the floor to support your body weight. Keeping your left knee on the floor, straighten your right leg and extend it behind your body just short of touching the floor.

Movement: Slowly raise your right leg as high as comfortably possible, keeping it straight throughout the move. Contract your glutes and then reverse direction, returning back to the start position. After performing the desired number of repetitions, repeat the process on your left. When the move becomes easy to perform, attach leg weights to your ankles for added resistance.

Tips:
1. *Keep your back slightly arched.* Rounding your back during exercise performance increases strain to the lumbar area and should be avoided at all costs. Make sure to keep your lower back tight and slightly hyperextended (arched), maintaining this position throughout the move.

2. *Don't twist your body.* The natural tendency to twist your body to the side as you perform a rep can place undue torque on your torso. Instead, keep your body square with the floor, making sure it remains still throughout the move.

3. *Avoid touching the floor with your foot.* All too frequently, people allow the foot of their working leg to rest on the floor at the start of this move. Doing so, however, removes tension from the glutes and thereby reduces the effectiveness of the exercise. In order to maintain constant tension on the target muscle, your toes should stop just short of touching the ground. This will maximize gluteal development.

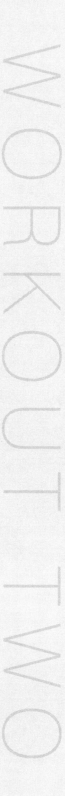

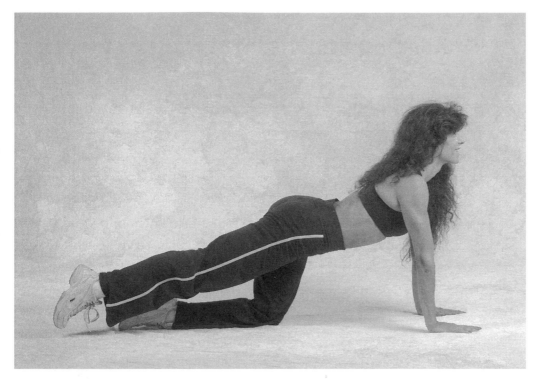

FIGURE 8.13 FLOOR KICK

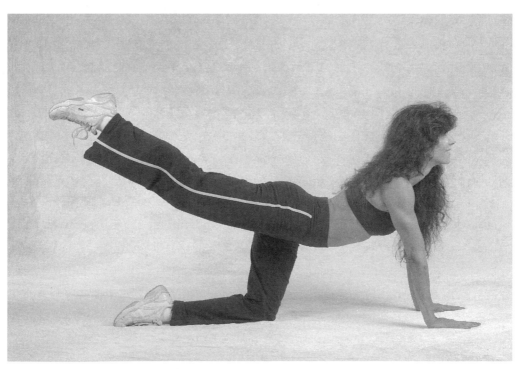

FIGURE 8.14 FLOOR KICK

SEATED HEEL RAISE

Target muscles: *Calves*

Secondary muscles used: *None*

Start: Sit on a bench or chair. Position a step (or block of wood) in front of your body and place your toes on the step, allowing your heels to descend as far as comfortably possible. Rest a dumbbell on your thighs and hold it in place.

Movement: Simultaneously raise your heels as high as possible, transferring your weight to the balls of your feet. Feel a contraction in your calf muscles and then slowly reverse direction, descending along the same path back to the start position.

Tips:

1. *Keep your feet pointed straight ahead.* Although some people believe that you can selectively target various portions of the calf muscles by altering foot position, this simply isn't the case. In actuality, extreme foot positions have contributed little to improving muscular shape and can readily cause damage to the ankle joint. For best results, keep your feet pointed straight ahead.

2. *Go slow on the negative.* While it is always imperative to remain in control on the negative (eccentric) portion of the repetition, this is especially true during calf training. As your heel lowers to the floor, you stretch your Achilles tendon, applying a great deal of force to this area. If you aren't careful, serious injury can occur to your Achilles tendon—a potentially disastrous event. Always lower slowly on the negative movement without bouncing and stretch only to the point that the muscle allows.

3. *Stretch your calves after your set.* Only one major artery feeds each of the calf muscles causing blood flow to be reduced to these muscles during training. This causes metabolic by-products such as lactic acid to accrue rapidly and increases the potential for muscular cramping. Stretching helps to flush the calves and decrease cramping, allowing better recuperation following training.

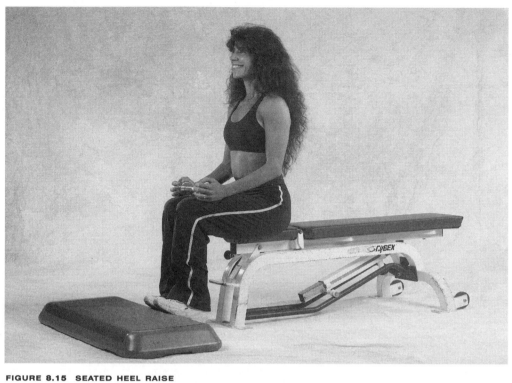

FIGURE 8.15 SEATED HEEL RAISE

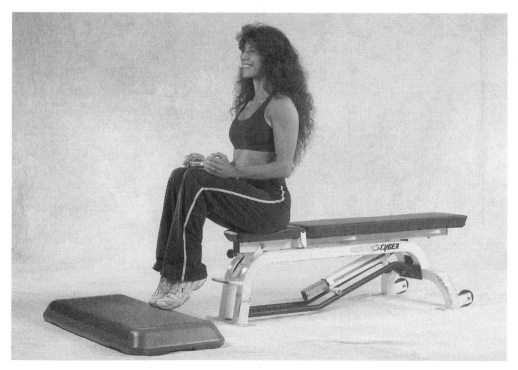

FIGURE 8.16 SEATED HEEL RAISE

WORKOUT TWO

REVERSE CURL

Target muscles: *Abdominals*

Secondary muscles used: *None*

Start: Lie back on the floor. Bring your knees into your stomach and keep your hands at your sides.

Movement: Slowly raise your butt as high as possible while keeping your upper back pressed to the floor. Contract your abs and then reverse direction, returning to the start position.

Tips:

1. *Don't use momentum.* Swinging your legs up in an effort to complete a rep takes stress away from the abs, diminishing muscular development. For best results, focus on achieving top-quality repetitions and don't worry if you are unable to reach your target rep range. Over time, your endurance will improve and the amount of reps that you can perform will increase.

2. *Your upper back must stay on the ground at all times.* There is a temptation to lift your upper back up on the eccentric (lowering) portion of the move to gain momentum during performance. This only serves to reduce tension in the lower abdominals. To perform the lift correctly, you must press your upper back into the floor and pull up only from the pelvis.

3. *When it becomes easy to perform the given number of reps, use a weight for added resistance.* There is little utility in performing more than twenty reps of any exercise. Doing so turns the move into an aerobic endeavor, diminishing gains in lean-muscle tissue. Thus, once you develop considerable abdominal strength, it is beneficial to wear leg weights during performance of the move.

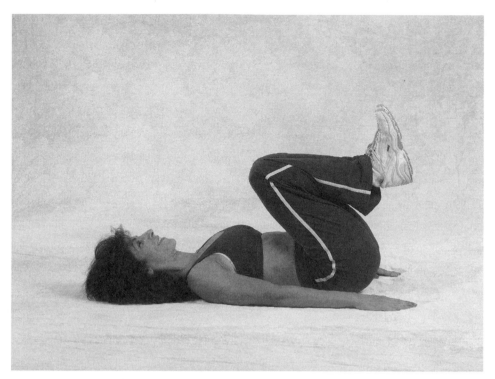

FIGURE 8.17 REVERSE CURL

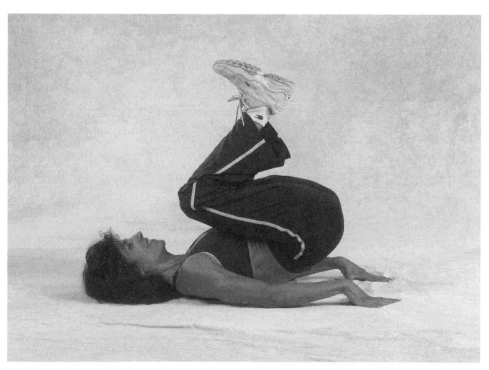

FIGURE 8.18 REVERSE CURL

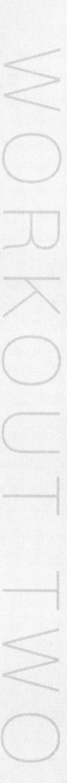

SUMMARY: WORKOUT TWO

Table 8.1 summarizes the specifics of Workout Two. Since everyone has different initial strength and fitness levels, you should use the suggested starting weights only as a guide and adjust them according to your individual strength levels. If you have never trained before and do not have someone who will supervise your workout and demonstrate proper exercise form, it can be beneficial to begin simply by learning the performance of each exercise without any weights. Do this as long as it takes to understand each movement.

Table 8.1

WORKOUT TWO					
MUSCLE GROUP	**EXERCISE**	**REPS**	**SETS**	**REST INTERVAL**	**STARTING WEIGHT**
CHEST	Incline Flye	15 to 20	1	30 Seconds	5
UPPER BACK	Dumbbell Pullover	15 to 20	1	30 Seconds	8
SHOULDERS	Arnold Press	15 to 20	1	30 Seconds	5
BICEPS	Incline Curl	15 to 20	1	30 Seconds	5
TRICEPS	Overhead Dumbbell Extension	15 to 20	1	30 Seconds	8
QUADRICEPS	Squat	15 to 20	1	30 Seconds	3
HAMS/GLUTES	Floor Kick	15 to 20	1	30 Seconds	No Weight
CALVES	Seated Heel Raise	15 to 20	1	30 Seconds	10
ABDOMINALS	Reverse Curl	15 to 20	1	30 Seconds	No Weight

CHAPTER 9

Workout Three

For Vilma Lusardi, balancing fitness with her busy work schedule is a chore. As a successful entrepreneur, she's constantly on the go. Compounding matters, her job is physically demanding. She makes her own brand of pasta sauce (healthy sauces, of course!) and, in the course of her marketing efforts, has to lug boxes of marinara around to various supermarkets and grocery stores throughout her area.

Vilma, 46, is a relative newbie to fitness. She started working out a mere five years ago. Her motives were simple: after turning forty, she realized that the only way to stave off the effects of aging was through exercise. And once the results manifested, she became hooked. Today, regardless of her commitments, she manages to train three days a week, even if she has to adjust her work schedule to do it.

While Vilma credits exercise for rejuvenating her body, she is most thankful for the strength increases it has provided. Before she started working out, Vilma needed help from her husband to lift many of the heavy items associated with her job. Now that's in the past—with her well-developed muscles, she's able to to it all on her own!

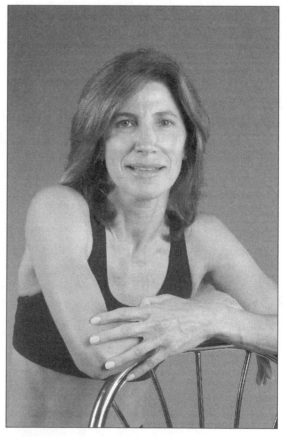

VILMA LUSARDI

WORKOUT THREE

MODIFIED PUSH-UP

Target muscles: *Chest*

Secondary muscles used: *Frontal shoulders and triceps*

Start: Begin with your hands and knees on the floor. Your torso should remain rigid, keeping your back perfectly straight throughout the move.

Movement: Bend your arms and slowly lower your body downward, stopping just before your upper chest touches the floor. Feel a stretch in your chest muscles and then reverse direction, pushing your body up along the same path back to the start position.

Tips:

1. *Don't allow your butt to drop down.* I commonly see people wiggle their entire bodies in an attempt to complete a push-up. They look like caterpillars as they try to get their bodies off the floor. It is important to keep your body on an even plane throughout the move. Your legs and torso should be perfectly straight, with all the movement happening at the arms.

2. *Don't let your elbows come close to your body.* Most women give little regard to the position of their arms during the performance of chest exercises. But when your elbows approach your sides, the chest muscles slacken, which leads to decreased results. To maintain tension on the chest, make sure your elbows flare out to the sides at all times. They should form a right angle with your body at the start of each rep.

3. *Alter the movement to suit your needs.* Since this exercise uses body weight for resistance, it can be difficult for some women to execute. If you have trouble with the movement, perform "half-reps," going only partway down. As time goes on, you'll be able to gradually increase the range of motion as you get stronger. Once the move becomes easy from a modified position, perform it "military style," with your lower body supported from your feet instead of your knees.

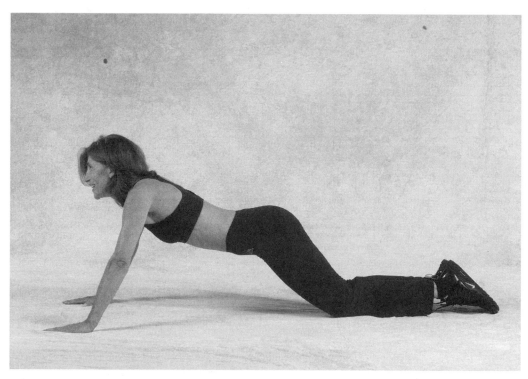

FIGURE 9.1 MODIFIED PUSH-UP

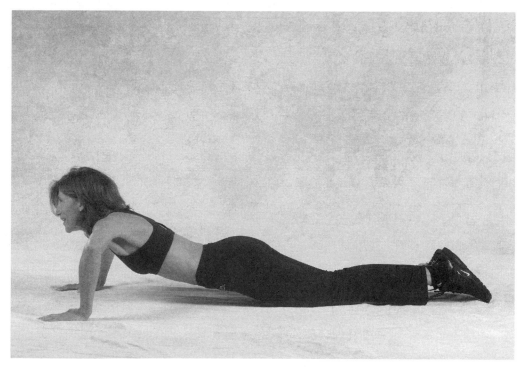

FIGURE 9.2 MODIFIED PUSH-UP

BENT DUMBBELL ROW

Target muscles: *Back*

Secondary muscles used: *Biceps and forearms*

Start: Bend your body forward and arch your lower back. Grasp a dumbbell in each hand and allow them to hang straight down from your shoulders with your palms facing your body.

Movement: Keeping your elbows close to your sides, pull the dumbbells upward as high as possible. Contract the muscles in your upper back and then slowly return the dumbbells back to the start position.

Tips:

1. *Don't round your back while lifting.* The tendency to round your back during performance, especially toward the end of a set, reduces the ability to contract the upper back muscles and places a great deal of stress on the lower back. Focus on keeping your lower back tight, maintaining a slight hyperextension during performance.

2. *Keep your elbows in.* When you swing your arms outward to pull up the weight, your shoulders and arms become increasingly active in the exercise. Your joints and connective tissue are also excessively stressed, heightening injury to this area. For best results, make sure that your elbows remain in as you execute the movement, keeping your upper arms close to your torso at all times.

3. *Make sure you achieve a full stretch at the bottom of the movement.* This is one of the few exercises during which you can lock out your elbow without ill effect. Doing so allows the muscles of the upper back to fully uncoil, promoting better development. In order to accentuate a stretch to this area, let the weight drift slightly forward on the descent.

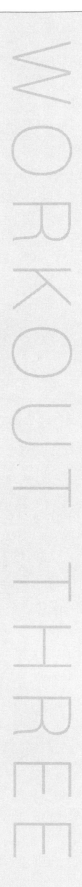

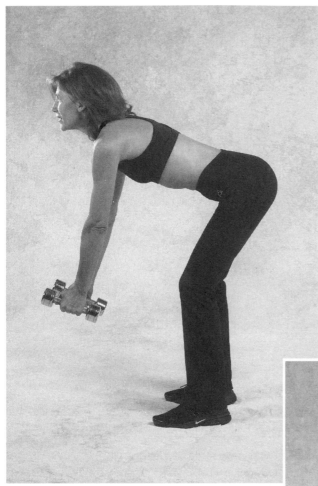

FIGURE 9.3   BENT DUMBBELL ROW

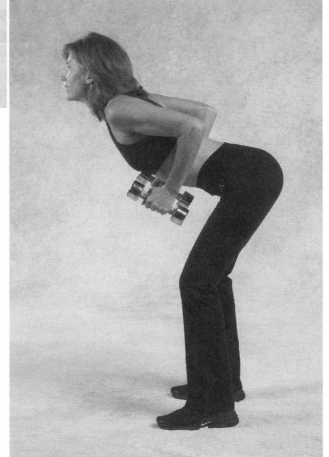

FIGURE 9.4   BENT DUMBBELL ROW

WORKOUT THREE

DUMBBELL UPRIGHT ROW

Target muscles: *Shoulders*

Secondary muscles used: *Upper back*

Start: Grasp a dumbbell in each hand and assume a shoulder-width, overhand grip. Allow your arms to hang down from your shoulders and assume a comfortable stance with your knees slightly bent.

Movement: Slowly bring the dumbbells upward along the line of your body until they approach your chin, keeping your elbows higher than your wrists at all times. Contract the muscles in your shoulders and then slowly return the dumbbells to the start position.

Tips:

1. *Pull from your elbows, not your hands.* A common error made in this move is to raise the hands upward during performance, especially when the shoulder muscles become fatigued. This only serves to involve the forearms, though, not the target muscles of the shoulders. As you lift, your hands should remain down at all times, below the plane of your shoulders. Remember, this is a shoulder exercise—not an arm exercise. Force the shoulder muscles to do the work!

2. *Don't shrug your shoulders at the top of the move.* During the execution of this movement, do not elevate the shoulders as the weights are lifted. This is counterproductive, as it overly involves your trapezius muscle and increases tension in your neck. Try to relax the shoulders as you perform the exercise, allowing only the muscles to do the work.

3. *Don't bring your upper arms above shoulder level.* It can be dangerous to lift the weights too high at the finish of the move. When abduction combined with internal rotation goes past 90 degrees, the greater tubercle (upper arm bone) approaches the acromium (part of the shoulder blade), which can impinge on the supraspinatus tendon and long head of the biceps. Hence, it is advisable to raise the elbows only to a point where the upper arms are parallel to the floor. This will ensure safe, effective performance.

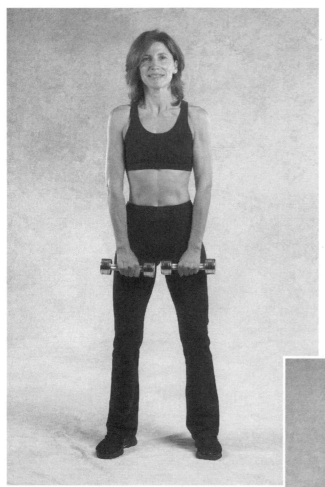

FIGURE 9.5 DUMBBELL UPRIGHT ROW

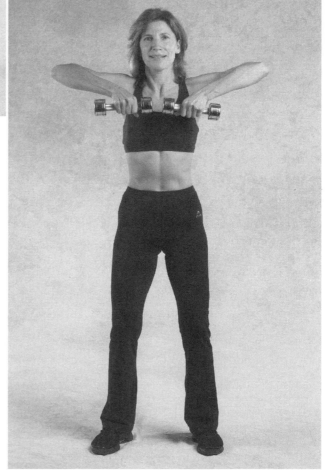

FIGURE 9.6 DUMBBELL UPRIGHT ROW

WORKOUT THREE

BENCH PREACHER CURL

Target muscles: *Biceps*

Secondary muscles used: *Forearms*

Start: Grasp a dumbbell with your right hand. Place the upper portion of your right arm on an incline bench and allow your right forearm to extend just short of locking the elbow.

Movement: Keeping your upper arm pressed to the bench, slowly curl the dumbbell upward toward your shoulders. Contract your biceps and then slowly return the weight to the start position. After completing the desired number of reps, repeat the process on your left.

Tips:

1. *Keep your wrists taut during the lift.* Since some women have weak wrists, maintaining stability in this area often becomes problematic. Consequently, during biceps movements, it is common to roll the wrists during performance. This removes stress from the biceps and transfers it to the muscles of the forearms. In order to counteract this effect, you must avoid letting your wrists bend downward, locking them in a fixed position throughout the move.

2. *Keep your upper arms in contact with the bench.* In an effort to get better leverage, there is a tendency to lift the upper arm up during performance. However, this decreases the involvement of the biceps. For best results, your upper arm should be pressed into the support pads of the bench at all times.

3. *Don't lock your elbows.* All too often, people completely straighten their arms at the start of this move. Locking your elbows not only takes stress away from the target muscle; it also makes the joint susceptible to injury. Accordingly, you should always maintain a slight elbow bend when lowering the weight.

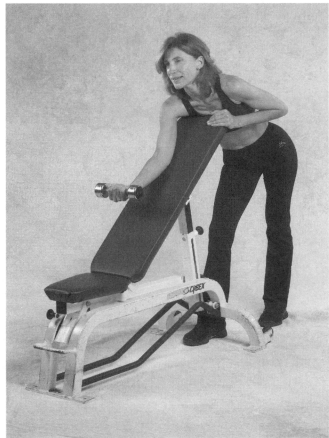

FIGURE 9.7 BENCH PREACHER CURL

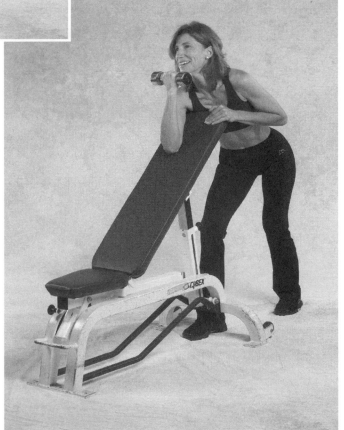

FIGURE 9.8 BENCH PREACHER CURL

TRICEPS DIP

Target muscles: *Triceps*

Secondary muscles used: *None*

Start: Place your feet on the floor and your hands on the edge of a flat bench. Keep your arms straight and your knees slightly bent.

Movement: Slowly bend your elbows as far as comfortably possible, allowing your butt to descend below the level of the bench. Make sure your elbows stay close to your body throughout the move. Then, reverse direction and straighten your arms, returning to the start position.

Tips:

   1. *Don't flare your elbows.* Elbow position is extremely important in all triceps extensions—but especially in dips. Allowing your arms to flare out brings the lats and chest muscles into play, taking stimulation away from the smaller triceps. It also places undue stress on the joints, potentially injuring the connective tissue. For best results, keep your elbows facing to the rear at all times and force your upper arms to remain close to your body as you rise up to the start position.

   2. *Alter the movement to suit your needs.* Since this exercise uses body weight for resistance, it can be difficult for some women to execute. If you have trouble with the movement, perform half-reps, going only partway down. As time goes on, you'll be able to increase the range of motion gradually as you get stronger.

   3. *Don't squirm around.* Shimmying your body to complete a rep removes stress from the triceps. Force your body to remain stable throughout the exercise, using only your arms to execute the movement.

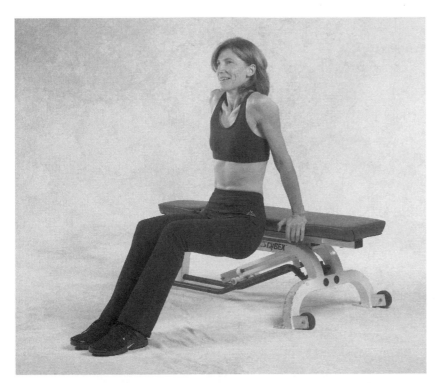

FIGURE 9.9   TRICEPS DIP

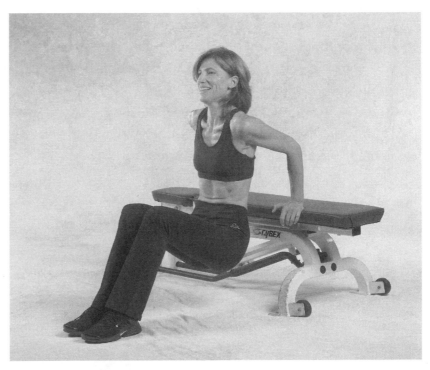

FIGURE 9.10   TRICEPS DIP

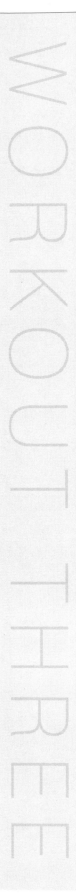

STEP UP

Target muscles: *Quadriceps*

Secondary muscles used: *Hamstrings and glutes*

Start: Grasp a dumbbell in each hand and allow them to hang at your sides. Stand facing the side of a flat bench with your feet shoulder-width apart.

Movement: Pushing off your right leg, step up with your left foot and follow with your right foot so that both feet are flat on the bench. Step back down in the same order, first with your left foot and then with your right, returning to the start position.

Tips:

1. *Use a moderate step height.* Weight benches come in various heights. An overly high bench can place an excessive strain on the joints, especially at the knee. A good rule of thumb is to have a step height that allows for hip flexion of no more than 90 degrees (the point where your thigh is parallel to the floor). In the beginning, you can start with a lower elevation and gradually increase step height as you gain strength.

2. *Don't rush the movement.* A cardinal rule of exercise is always to be in control (remember the ABCs of lifting!). Nowhere is this more important than in the step up. Going too fast can easily cause you to lose your balance and fall. Thus, make sure you proceed at a deliberate pace, and step in the middle of the bench on each rep.

3. *Keep your toes pointed straight ahead.* Rotating your feet too far in either direction can not only turn your ankle, but also can cause severe injury to your knee joint. For best results, your toes should remain within 15 degrees of forward.

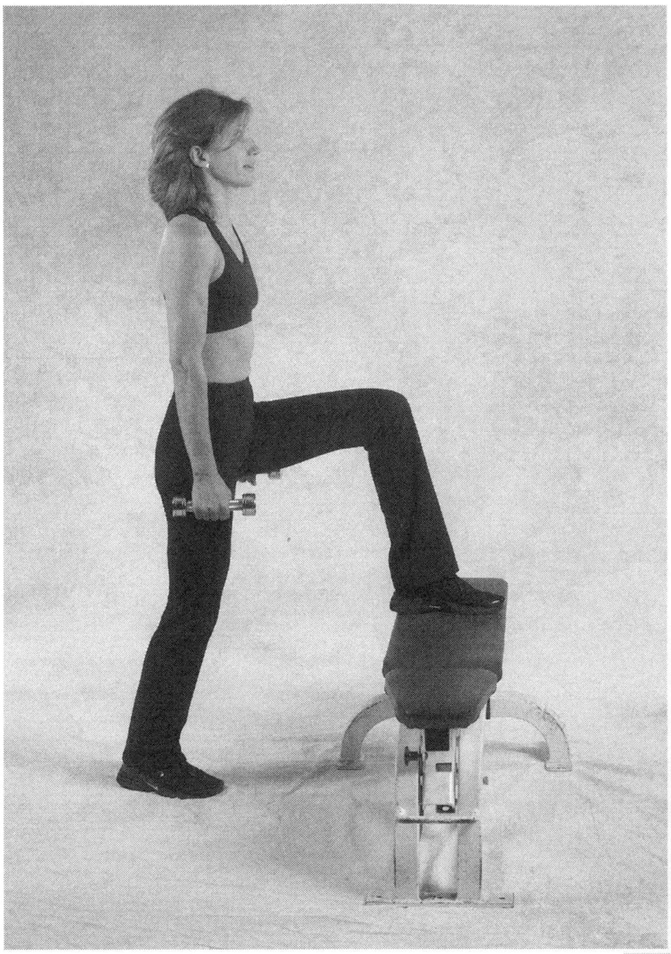

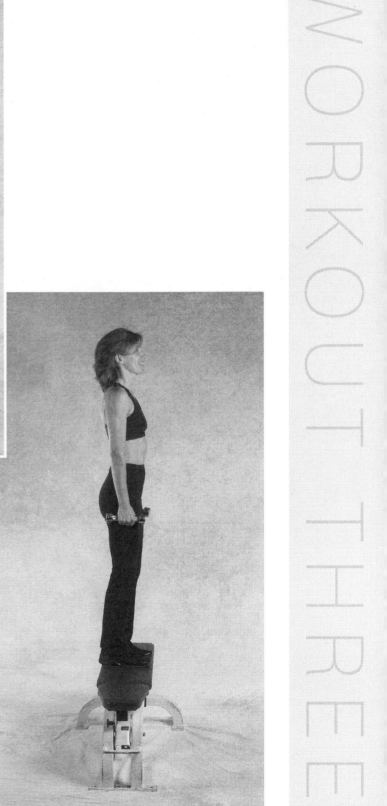

FIGURE 9.11 STEP UP

FIGURE 9.12 STEP UP

WORKOUT THREE

PRONE BODY RAISE

Target muscles: *Hamstrings, glutes*

Secondary muscles used: *Lower back*

Start: Lie facedown on the floor or a mat. Keep your feet together and allow your arms to rest at your sides.

Movement: Simultaneously raise your shoulders and legs off the ground as high as comfortably possible, making sure that your head remains stable throughout the move. Contract your glutes and then reverse direction, returning to the start position.

Tips:

1. *Don't lift from the neck.* Extending the neck as you raise your body from the floor can easily strain the soft tissues of the cervical spine. Rather, make sure that your neck is stationary through-out the move. The action should take place only at the torso.

2. *Don't overextend the lower back.* If you lift your torso too far off the floor, the muscles of the lower back can become overstressed, causing injury to the region. The goal should be to achieve a muscular contraction without feeling strain in the area. Everyone has varying degrees of flexibility. Stay within your range.

3. *Don't twist your body.* When you lift your torso, any twisting motion can result in an injury, especially to your obliques (the muscles on the side of your body). This is especially pertinent when you get fatigued and struggle to complete the last few reps of a set. Therefore, it is important to lift straight up, without pulling toward one side.

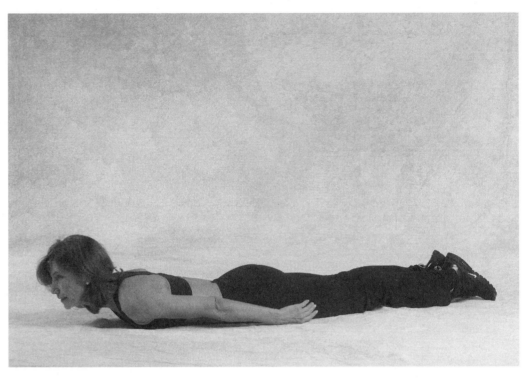

FIGURE 9.13   PRONE BODY RAISE

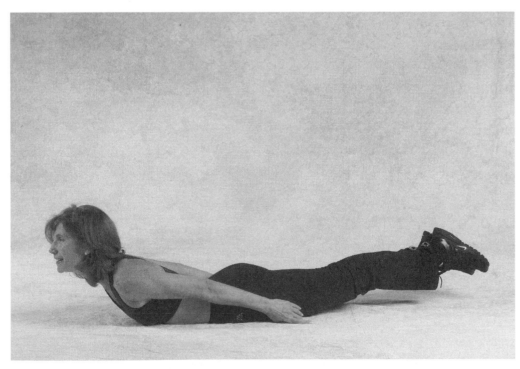

FIGURE 9.14   PRONE BODY RAISE

ONE-LEGGED HEEL RAISE

Target muscles: *Calves*

Secondary muscles used: *None*

Start: Stand upright and grasp a dumbbell in your left hand. Hold on to a stationary object for support with your right hand and bend your right knee so that your lower leg is behind your body.

Movement: Simultaneously raise your left heel as high as possible, transferring your weight to the ball of your foot. Feel a contraction in your calf muscle and then slowly reverse direction, descending along the same path back to the start position. After finishing the required number of repetitions, repeat on the opposite side.

Tips:

1. *Don't lean forward during the move.* Do not tilt to the front as your heel is elevated. This can cause you to lose balance and fall forward. Therefore, keep your body completely erect as you ascend, centering your weight so that balance is maintained.

2. *Go slow on the negative.* It is imperative that you remain in control on the negative (eccentric) portion of the repetition. As your heel lowers to the floor, you stretch your Achilles tendon, applying a great deal of force to this area. If you aren't careful, serious injury can occur to your Achilles tendon. Always lower slowly on the negative movement without bouncing and stretch only to the point that the muscle allows.

3. *Perform the move on stairs for increased resistance.* Once you can easily perform the target number of repetitions, challenge yourself by executing the move on the bottom step of a staircase. By placing your foot on the edge of the step, you can allow your heel to stretch down, significantly increasing your range of motion. In this version, make sure to hold on to the banister for support.

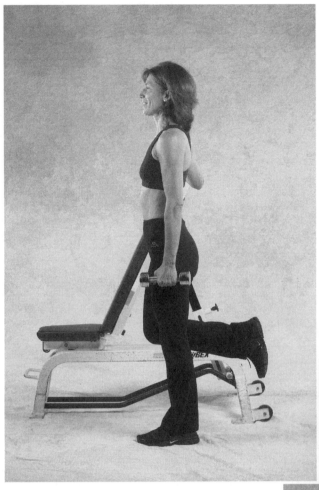

FIGURE 9.15 ONE-LEGGED HEEL RAISE

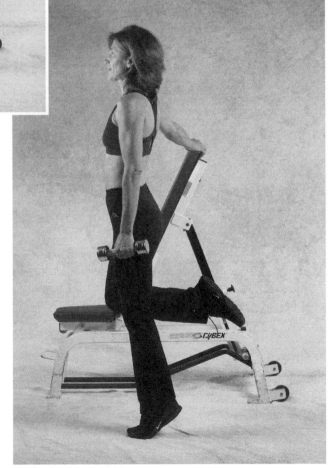

FIGURE 9.16 ONE-LEGGED HEEL RAISE

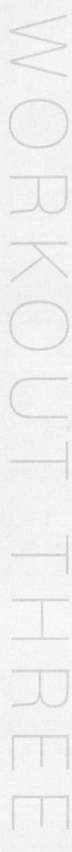

SIDE JACKKNIFE

Target muscles: *Abdominals*

Secondary muscles used: *None*

Start: Lie on your left side with your right leg in the air. Make a fist with your right hand and keep it pressed to your right ear.

Movement: Raise your torso upward as far as possible so that your elbow approaches your leg. Contract your oblique muscles and then slowly reverse direction and return to the start position. After performing the prescribed number of repetitions, repeat the process on the left.

Tips:

1. *Don't flex your torso too far.* In an effort to bring the elbow as close to the leg as possible, some people push their muscles too far. This invariably causes a soft-tissue injury. Remember, everyone has different degrees of flexibility. If you can touch your elbow to your leg, great; if not, don't worry. Just bring your torso up as far as you can.

2. *Don't lift from your leg.* Lifting the leg during the course of the move will confer no benefit on your oblique muscles. For maximal results, all the movement must take place at the waist.

3. *Keep your head stable.* Allowing the neck to move sideways during exercise performance can easily strain the cervical muscles. To avoid this fate, make sure that your neck remains immobile throughout the move.

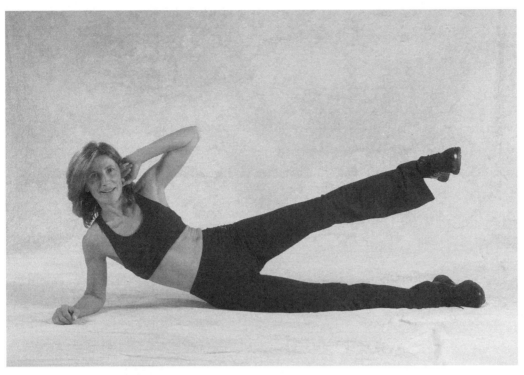

FIGURE 9.17 SIDE JACKKNIFE

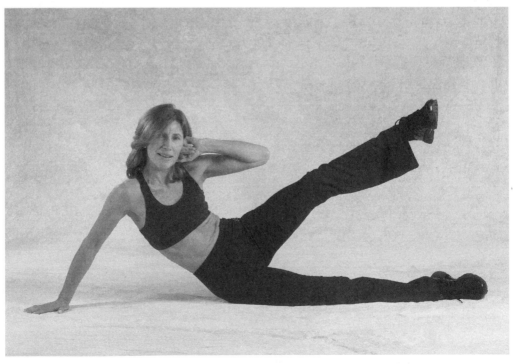

FIGURE 9.18 SIDE JACKKNIFE

WORKOUT THREE

SUMMARY: WORKOUT THREE

Table 9.1 summarizes the specifics of Workout Three. Since everyone has different initial strength and fitness levels, you should use the suggested starting weights only as a guide and adjust them according to your individual strength levels. If you have never trained before and do not have someone who will supervise your workout and demonstrate proper exercise form, it can be beneficial to begin simply by learning the performance of each exercise without any weights. Do this as long as it takes to understand each movement.

Table 9.1

WORKOUT THREE					
MUSCLE GROUP	**EXERCISE**	**REPS**	**SETS**	**REST INTERVAL**	**STARTING WEIGHT**
CHEST	Push-up	15	1	30 Seconds	No Weight
UPPER BACK	Bent Dumbbell Row	15	1	30 Seconds	5
SHOULDERS	Upright Row	15	1	30 Seconds	5
BICEPS	Bench Preacher Curl	15	1	30 Seconds	5
TRICEPS	Triceps Dip	15	1	30 Seconds	No Weight
QUADRICEPS	Step Up	15	1	30 Seconds	3
HAMS/GLUTES	Prone Body Raise	15	1	30 Seconds	No Weight
CALVES	One-Legged Standing Heel Raise	15	1	30 Seconds	5
ABDOMINALS	Side Jackknife	15	1	30 Seconds	No Weight

THE NUTRITION FACTOR

PART THREE

CHAPTER 10

Eat to Your Health

L ose thirty pounds in thirty days . . ."

"Take two inches off your waist in two weeks . . ."

"Drop a dress size this weekend . . ."

Anyone who watches television, listens to the radio, or reads magazines has undoubtedly heard these types of claims for "magic diets" promising an easy way to shed unwanted pounds. We live in a society that craves instant gratification, and the prospect of achieving a rapid physical transformation is hard to resist. After all, wouldn't it be great to leave work on a Friday and come back Monday morning looking like a new person? Legions of struggling dieters sure think so!

The truth is "magic diets" don't really work. While most of these programs will induce temporary weight loss, they simply don't provide the ability to sustain results over the long haul. They are short-term solutions to a long-term problem and neglect to teach proper eating patterns. This is the primary reason why fewer than 10 percent of those who go on a diet are able to keep the weight off after just a year's time.

Ketogenic (i.e., low-carb) diets are notorious for causing rapid weight loss—as much as fifteen pounds in the first two weeks. Most of the weight loss, though, is from water—not body fat. The reason is simple: Glycogen, the stored form of carbohydrate, is hydrophilic (water loving). For each gram of glycogen, the body stores about three grams of water. Hence, when carbs are eliminated from the diet, diuresis (fluid loss) is encouraged causing the kidneys to excrete water. But these effects are short-lived. As soon as a ketogenic diet is discontinued and carbs are reintroduced into your system, all the water weight returns.

The problem with any extreme diet is that there is not only a reduction of fat, but of lean tissue, as well. When calories are severely restricted, up to 45 percent of the energy deficit is derived from burning muscle for fuel—a fact that can account for as much as one pound a week of muscle loss. This muscle loss causes an associated drop in your metabolism making it increasingly difficult to lose body fat as time goes by. In the end, regained weight is almost always higher than it was before dieting.

DEVELOPING A STRATEGY

It is important to realize that there is no single "best" diet. Every woman has a unique nutritional profile and, based on a host of genetic and lifestyle factors, responds differently to various foods. Things such as metabolic rate, insulin sensitivity, and activity level all influence dietary requirements. Therefore, it is unrealistic to follow a cookie-cutter nutritional prescription and expect it to work for you. Chances are, your specific needs won't be adequately addressed.

The key to promoting long-term, sustainable weight management is to develop a sound nutritional strategy that becomes a way of life. An effective program balances caloric intake with caloric expenditure, stabilizes insulin, and increases metabolism. It must be sensible as well as practical. My approach to nutrition combines all these facets and is based on nutritional science—not gimmicks. It is specific in its recommendations, yet it is flexible enough to be adapted to your individual needs. Whether you want to lose, gain, or maintain your current weight, this program will help you achieve your goals.

The guiding principle behind my nutritional program is the law of thermodynamics: If you take in more calories than you expend, you'll gain weight; if you take in fewer calories than you expend, you'll lose weight; and if intake and expenditure are in equilibrium, your weight will remain stable. Despite claims of various "diet gurus," this concept is immutable.

LOSING WEIGHT

For safe, effective weight loss, a maximum of one to two pounds can be lost per week. But the important thing to focus on is fat loss, not weight loss—remember, you don't want to lose precious muscle tissue! The first step in this process is to figure out your daily caloric maintenance level (DCML): the number of calories required each day to maintain a stable body weight. A simple way to estimate DCML is to multiply your body weight by 14 (body weight × 14). Thus, a woman who weighs 150 pounds would need approximately 3,100 calories to maintain her current weight. While this formula only provides a crude approximation of daily caloric intake, it at least gives you a starting point from which to work. From here, modifications can be made based on your individual needs.

To induce fat loss, your DCML must be adjusted so that you expend more calories than you consume. This is simple mathematics. You can eat all the "right" foods, but if you take in too many calories from these foods, weight gain is inevitable. For example, consuming as few as 100 extra calories a day—the amount found in a handful of nachos or a dozen French fries—can result in a yearly weight gain of more than ten pounds! Only by creating a caloric deficit is it possible to lose body fat.

When you first begin reducing calories, it is best to be conservative. Start out with a 500-calorie reduction in your DCML and then gradually increase this amount if necessary. Just make sure to take it slow. A loss of one pound per week might not seem like a lot, but over the course of a year, it equates to a 52-pound drop! Remember, rapid weight loss will only serve to sabotage your long-term fitness goals. If you experience a loss of more than two pounds in a week, increase your caloric intake accordingly to stay in the prescribed range.

MACRONUTRIENT PROFILE

Once you have determined your caloric intake, you must now focus on the percentage of calories that will be derived from carbohydrates, protein, and fat—the so-called "macronutrients." To get the most out of your diet, it is imperative that you take in the right mix of these nutrients. All calories are not the same, and each nutrient has specific functions and affects the body in different ways. Let's discuss how these nutrients should be apportioned for optimal benefits.

Carbohydrates

Carbohydrates aren't the enemy! No matter what you may have heard, simply cutting out carbs from your diet won't miraculously induce fat loss or help you maintain ideal health and wellness. In fact, ketogenic diets can actually impair your body composition over the long haul.

Although not essential for life function, carbohydrates are integrally involved in many bodily processes. They help to preserve tissue proteins, assist in fat metabolism, and stoke the central nervous system.

From a weight-management perspective, there's good reason to eat carbohydrates. You see, carbs increase production of triiodothyronine (T3), a primary thyroid hormone that is integrally involved in the regulation of metabolic rate. A low carb intake can compromise thyroid function and thereby suppress metabolism. Thus, to keep your body's cellular furnace running at peak efficiency, it's important to include a healthy dose of carbs in your diet.

Carbs are particularly important as you exercise. The compounds derived from carbohydrate breakdown are stored as glycogen in your muscles and liver. Glycogen is the primary fuel used to power your muscles during intense workouts. It provides an instant source of energy that can be accessed on demand, enabling you to train at a high level of intensity.

When carbohydrate intake is severely restricted, your body has to convert amino acids into glucose (through a process called *gluconeogenesis*) in order to meet short-term energy needs. However, this conversion process is very inefficient and fails to supply an adequate amount of energy reserves. Ultimately, your stamina begins to wane and you soon become lethargic and irritable. Complications including nausea, and headaches and dizziness are apt to occur. There is a degradation in exercise performance, diminishing your ability to develop lean muscle tone. Overall, your physical and mental fitness becomes compromised.

With this in mind, it's important to understand that all carbs are not alike. Standard nutritional advice has always been to eat "complex" carbs and avoid "simple" ones, based on the belief that simple carbs have a negative effect on insulin while complex carbs are "insulin friendly." Given the detriments associated with an oversecretion of insulin, the preference for complex carbs certainly seems justified.

In reality, though, carbohydrates don't always behave according to their complexity. For instance, it has been determined that many complex carbs like potatoes and white bread actually cause a large insulin response while simple carbs such as apples and oranges don't. This turns the whole complex-carb theory on its head.

A better mode of carbohydrate classification is based on the glycemic index. Originally created to help diabetics adjust their insulin dosage, the glycemic index ranks foods on how they affect blood-sugar levels. By measuring the speed at which carbs enter the bloodstream, it provides a reasonably accurate indication of their impact on insulin secretion. Carbs that cause a rapid elevation of blood sugar (glucose) are termed high glycemic, while those that are "time released" and maintain stable levels of blood sugar are called low glycemic.

As a rule, refined, sugar-laden foods are high glycemic, as they are rapidly absorbed into circulation, causing a spike in your blood-sugar levels. Consequently, your pancreas secretes large quantities of insulin as a means to clear the sugar from your bloodstream. This excess insulin is directly responsible for converting sugars into body fat as well as inhibiting the conversion of stored fat into energy. This double whammy greatly increases the potential for body-fat storage.

Excess insulin also removes sugars from your circulatory system in such an expeditious fashion that there is a dramatic drop in blood-sugar levels. A hypoglycemic state ensues, causing severe hunger pangs and food cravings. This creates a vicious cycle that encourages binge eating—especially of sweets. The cycle goes around and around, inevitably leading to gains in fat mass.

Conversely, unrefined grains tend to be low glycemic. These foods are broken down more slowly by the body. They enter the bloodstream in a time-released fashion, keeping blood-sugar levels in check. As a result, insulin is released gradually into your system, reducing the activity of fat-storing enzymes and therefore helping to maintain a lean physique. In fact, it has been shown that simply substituting simple sugars with lower-glycemic carbohydrates reduces the amount of fat storage—all without changing the total number of calories consumed!

Consuming low-glycemic carbs also helps to enhance energy levels. Because of their slow entry into circulation, glucose, an instant fuel source, is available for an extended time period. Glucose allows your muscles to perform vigorous activity and promotes optimal brain function. With a steady stream of glucose from which to draw, your physical and mental acuity remains at its peak throughout the day.

It is best to keep consumption of high-glycemic foods—especially refined sugars—to an absolute minimum. When eaten in abundance, they can be one of the biggest obstacles to maintaining a lean, fit physique. A good rule of thumb is to "think brown" when eating starches instead of choosing "white" starches. For example, replace potatoes with yams, white rice with brown rice, refined pasta with the whole-wheat variety, and plain bread with seven-grain bread. These low-glycemic alternatives will keep blood sugar in check and stabilize insulin secretions, which will minimize fat storage.

RECOMMENDED INTAKE

Carbs should comprise approximately 40 to 50 percent of the calories in your diet. Unless you are an endurance athlete, any more than this amount is superfluous. Start out on the low end of the spectrum, keeping carbs at the suggested minimum. If you feel lethargic or fatigued, increase your carb intake by another 5 percent. If you still don't have enough energy, take carbs up to the maximum.

Green vegetables should constitute a significant portion of carb intake. On a volume basis, they are extremely low in calories and high in nutritional value. Think of them as green water—they can be consumed in large amounts without making you fat. A pound of broccoli, for instance, contains only about 120 calories (compare that to a pound of pasta, which has about 1,600 calories!). Because of their bulk, they take up a large amount of space in the stomach, which helps to suppress food cravings, preventing the urge to overeat. And considering that they are replete with vitamins and minerals, green vegetables should be a staple in your diet.

Fiber

Although not a "macronutrient" per se, fiber plays an important role in overall nutrition. Fiber is unique in that it cannot be completely digested and passes down directly into the colon unimpeded. This means that fiber has virtually no caloric value; its consumption can't make you gain weight!

There is a large body of scientific evidence indicating that a diet high in fiber is beneficial to your health. At the very least, it helps to maintain bowel regularity. Because fiber absorbs water in the large intestine, it causes your stools to become soft and fluffy, thereby preventing constipation. The increase in stool volume also helps to dilute the concentration of bile acids, which are thought to instigate the growth of malignant tumors. Studies have shown that a diet high in fiber can result in up to a 30 percent reduction in these malignancies, making it a potent cancer-fighting agent.

In addition, fiber consumption can cause a substantial decline in serum cholesterol levels. Reductions of up to 13 percent have been reported, with favorable effects on the ratio of "good" to "bad" cholesterol (HDL to LDL). Each 1 percent drop in cholesterol translates into a 2 percent drop in the risk of developing heart disease.

Besides having a positive effect on your well-being, fiber also plays an important role in weight management. Fiber forms a "gel" in the intestines, inhibiting the digestion and absorption of nutrients. As food passes through your intestines, some of the nutrients get trapped in the gel and end up being excreted before they can be metabolized. Hence, you can eat more food without having it stored in your system. In fact, it has been reported that by simply doubling fiber intake from 18 to 36 grams, you reduce the available calories in your diet by more than 100 calories per day!

Fiber is found in a wide array of carb-based foods, especially unrefined grains, fruits, and vegetables. Appendix A shows some of the more popular high-fiber foods that you should consume readily as well as their corresponding fiber content. By maintaining a high-fiber diet, you'll go a long way toward improving your health as well as your body.

RECOMMENDED INTAKE

Fiber intake should exceed 20 grams per 1,000 calories consumed, with a minimum of 30 grams per day. This should be derived from a variety of fiber-rich foods to ensure that you get adequate amounts of both soluble and insoluble sources. If, for any reason, you have trouble getting enough fiber from whole foods, consider taking one of the many fiber supplements on the market. They are quick and convenient, allowing you to fiber up without a great deal of hassle.

Fat

Traditional wisdom has always taught that if you want to maintain a lean physique, dietary fat should be kept to a bare minimum. For many years, the majority of sports nutritionists emphatically stated, "Eat fat and you'll get fat!" A legion of health-conscious consumers listened, and zero-fat diets soon became the rage.

The problem with this theory, though, is that fats are an essential nutrient and play a vital role in many bodily functions. They are involved in cushioning your internal organs for protection, aiding in the absorption of vitamins, and facilitating the production of cell membranes, hormones, and prostaglandins. Physiologically, it would be impossible to survive without the inclusion of fats in your diet.

It is the "type" of fat—rather than fat, per se—that should be scrutinized from a dietary perspective. You see, fats are classified into two basic categories: saturated and unsaturated. Saturated fats, abundant in many meats and dairy products, remain solid at room temperature. For all intents and purposes, they serve no biological purpose. If not used immediately for energy, they either are stored in fat cells throughout your body or raise LDL levels and become oxidized as fatty deposits in your arteries. Over time, a large intake of these "bad" fats results in plaque buildup in your arteries, which ultimately can lead to a heart attack or stroke. Studies indicate there is a strong correlation between saturated-fat intake and cardiovascular mortality.

But that's not all. Studies have also shown that the consumption of saturated fats tends to make your muscles less responsive to insulin and inhibits your body's ability to store sugars as glycogen. This predisposes a person to insulin resistance, which, as previously discussed, results in a plethora of negative effects on well-being.

All things considered, you must keep your consumption of saturated fats to an absolute minimum. Fortunately, with a little nutritional savvy, they can be all but eliminated from your diet (see Table 10.1).

Unsaturated fats are healthier fats. As opposed to the saturated variety, these fats remain liquid at room temperature. Because of their fluid structure, they are quite biologically active and can interact in various systemic processes. This allows them to be readily utilized as a fuel source. While saturated fats tend to be stored in fat tissue, unsaturated fats are preferentially oxidized for energy. The implications are clear: all things being equal, saturated fats make you fatter than unsaturated fats.

Olive oil, a monounsaturated fat, is often called a "neutral" fat because it neither raises nor lowers blood-cholesterol levels. This, however, is somewhat misleading. Olive oil contains heart-healthy compounds such as phytosterols, polyphenols, and antioxidants that have been shown to improve lipid profiles. Hence, olive oil does indeed promote heart-healthy benefits.

When choosing an olive oil, make sure to get one that is "extra virgin." This ensures that it is completely unrefined and hasn't gone through industrial processes like degumming, bleaching, and deodorizing. These procedures remove the health-related benefits of the oil and render it nutritionally unsound.

The most important types of unsaturated fats from a dietary perspective are called essential fatty acids (EFAs). There are two basic types of EFAs: omega-3 and omega-6. These fats are polyunsatu-

Table 10.1

TIPS FOR REDUCING SATURATED FATS

1. Foods should be baked, broiled, steamed, or microwaved. Never fry foods.
2. Prepare your foods "dry," without using lard, oil, or butter in your cooking.
3. Trim all visible fat from your meats. Even lean cuts of meat normally have fat around the edges. Any fat that can be seen by the naked eye should be removed.
4. Remove the skin from poultry products. Do this *before* cooking since heat causes animal fat to seep into the meat.

rated (they contain two or more double bonds, as opposed to monounsaturates, which have only one) and, due to an absence of specific enzymes, cannot be manufactured by your body. Consequently, EFAs are an "essential" component in food; a deficiency ultimately causes a breakdown in cellular function.

EFAs have numerous healthful benefits. When consumed in moderation, they can actually expedite fat loss. This is accomplished in two ways. First, EFAs help to suppress two enzymes, fatty acid synthase and lipoprotein lipase, both of which are integrally involved in fat storage. Second, EFAs increase levels of a fat-burning protein called UCP (uncoupling protein). UCP acts on various bodily tissues, allowing calories to be burned off immediately as heat (a process known as thermogenesis) rather than stored as fat. The net effect of this dual combination is better fat metabolism and therefore improved body composition.

EFAs—especially omega-3 fatty acids—also have a cardioprotective effect, making them a "heart-healthy" nutrient. They inhibit the production of LDL (the "bad" form of cholesterol that has been implicated in the formation of anterial plaques) and increase the output of HDL (the "good" cholesterol, which scavenges LDL and returns it to the liver for excretion). Not only do EFAs help to prevent plaque buildup in otherwise healthy individuals, but they can even reverse arterial damage in those with existing heart disease. In fact, replacing saturated fats with EFAs has been shown to reduce the risk of mortality in those who have had heart attacks by as much as 70 percent!

The best sources of EFAs are found in soy products and deep-colored, cold-water fish such as salmon, mackerel, and tuna. They are also abundant in a variety of oils including flaxseed, rapeseed, safflower, and sunflower. These oils come in liquid form and can either be mixed into your foods or taken by the spoonful. An important consideration, though: EFAs cannot be used in cooking. Excessive heat breaks the unique double-bond structure of the unsaturated fat and makes it rancid. Vitamins and minerals literally go up in smoke, as do antioxidants. Toxic carcinogens are formed that wreak havoc on your cells, and all the benefits of EFAs are lost.

If you must cook with a fat-based product (it's best to prepare your foods "dry" if at all possible), you should do so with saturated fats such as butter, coconut oil, or palm oil. Since these fats contain no double bonds, they are quite stable even at high temperatures. Alternatively, oils such as grapeseed extract and canola oil have a high smoke point and tend to hold up relatively well under low levels of heat (such as stir-frying).

There is one type of unsaturated fat—called "trans fats"—that should be completely avoided. Although technically unsaturated, trans fats actually behave very much like saturated fats. They are formed during a process in which vegetable oils are heated and exposed to hydrogen gas. This process, called *partial hydrogenation*, solidifies the oil, giving it certain desirable qualities for cooking—namely spreadability and increased shelf life. However, with the good also comes the bad: Partial hydrogenation also destroys the healthy double-carbon bonds of the oil, producing compounds that are foreign to the human body.

From a cardiovascular standpoint, trans fats can be considered the "anti-EFAs." Their consumption has been shown to elevate blood levels of LDL (the "bad" cholesterol) and lower levels of HDL (the "good" cholesterol), which wreaks havoc on your arteries, making trans fats an even greater health-related detriment than saturated fats.

Trans fats are found in a wide array of processed foods. Margarine is perhaps the biggest culprit, with a whopping 60 percent of calories attributed to these unhealthy oils. Salad dressings, doughnuts, potato chips, and cookies all tend to have high amounts, as do many fast-food items such as French fries and chicken nuggets.

Unfortunately, it sometimes can be difficult to identify foods that contain trans fats because they are not listed separately on food labels. The best way to ensure that you avoid these villains is to check the ingredients. Stay away from anything that lists "partially hydrogenated" in the ingredients—especially if it is one of the first items mentioned. This indicates a food has a high trans-fat content and thus should be summarily avoided.

RECOMMENDED INTAKE

As a rule, limit your fat intake to approximately 20 percent of your total calories, with the majority coming from unsaturated sources—particularly EFAs. Ideally, the ratio of polyunsaturated fats to monounsaturated fats should be about 1:1. A good case can be made for consuming an even greater amount of polyunsaturates (particularly omega-3 fatty acids) due to their beneficial effects on body composition and cardiovascular health.

Despite the recent prominence of high-fat diets, excess fat consumption will almost certainly have a negative long-term impact on your health and body. Since virtually no energy is expended in their digestion, fats are more easily stored as body fat than any other nutrient. While proteins and carbs have a thermic effect on the body, the percentage of calories expended in the breakdown of fat is minimal.

Moreover, fats are dense with calories. Each gram of fat has 9 calories, as compared to carbohydrates and protein, which have only 4. Hence, a small portion of a fat-laden food has a much higher amount of calories than a comparable portion of a low-fat food. For example, a tablespoon of lard contains approximately 120 calories, while it takes about a pound of green beans to equal this amount! And since a large quantity of fatty foods is required to fill your stomach, the potential for overeating is dramatically increased.

Protein

Without question, protein is the king of all nutrients. It provides the raw materials for enzymes and hormones, enables nerve and brain cells to communicate effectively with one another, and fosters the repair and growth of muscle tissue. Since the body cannot manufacture protein internally, it must be obtained from dietary sources; life could not go on without it.

For active individuals, the need for protein is heightened. When you exercise, your body draws from a "pool" of amino acids—the building blocks of protein—for fuel. The branched-chain amino acids (BCAAs), in particular, are preferentially mobilized as an energy source during intense training. Consequently, by the end of an intense workout, there is a net degradation of amino acids—a fact that can only be rectified by consuming adequate dietary protein. If these amino acids aren't replenished, the body is unable to repair its muscle effectively and the quality of your physique suffers.

A diet high in protein has other benefits. Of all the macronutrients, protein is least likely to cause fat storage. Consider that a large percentage of calories from protein is burned off in the digestion process—a phenomenon called the *thermic effect of food*. Of all the macronutrients, protein has the highest thermic effect, burning off approximately 25 percent of the calories consumed. In comparison, only 10 percent of the calories from carbs are burned off in digestion; fat has virtually no thermic effect whatsoever.

What's more, protein tends to curb appetite. This is largely a hormonal function. When protein is consumed, a hormone called cholecystokinin (CCK) is secreted. Through an action that is not completely understood, CCK acts on the body's hunger mechanisms, quelling the urge to eat. Given the law of thermodynamics, these appetite-suppressing effects alone help to promote weight loss.

There is a widespread fallacy, though, that high-protein diets can be harmful to your health. This myth is based on the contention that a surplus of protein has a detrimental effect on kidney function. During digestion, protein is broken down into its component parts—the amino acids—via a process called deamination. A by-product of this occurrence is the production of ammonia—a toxic substance—in the body. But ammonia doesn't stay in the body for long; it is rapidly converted into the relatively nontoxic substance urea, which is then transported to the kidneys for excretion.

However, a large buildup of urea can overtax the kidneys (even though it is nontoxic), impairing their ability to carry out vital functions, especially for those with renal disease. It has been well documented that a high-protein diet exacerbates uremia (kidney failure) in those on dialysis; in direct contrast, a low-protein diet helps to alleviate the condition. If you have existing kidney damage, protein consumption should be kept to a minimum.

But in those with normal renal function, there is no evidence that a diet high in protein has any detrimental consequences. While increased protein intake does bring about some minor alterations in renal size and function, they are merely normal adaptations that aren't associated with any adverse effects. The consensus is that healthy kidneys are readily able to filter out urea; any excess is simply expelled in the urine.

So what are the best protein sources? Well, many terrific options exist—enough to satisfy almost everyone's taste buds. Here is a list of the top choices:

Poultry

Poultry is a protein powerhouse. Turkey and chicken, in particular, have long been favorites of bodybuilders and other physique-oriented athletes. But there is one caveat: You should only eat the white meat. The dark meat (found primarily in the drumsticks and wings) is actually extremely fatty, containing about as much saturated fat as chuck steak. So when shopping for poultry, make sure that the meat comes from the breast. This is especially important when buying ground poultry; eating a turkey burger made from dark meat is no healthier than eating a regular hamburger!

Seafood

Seafood is another great protein source. Many types of fish (such as flounder, cod, and grouper) are virtually devoid of any fat. Others (especially the cold-water variety such as salmon, mackerel, and trout) contain ample amounts of healthy EFAs—fats that are beneficial to health and well being. Either way, seafood gives you high-quality protein without tangibly increasing consumption of saturated fat. Better yet, it also provides a great deal of nutritional diversity. Each species of fish has its own unique taste and can be prepared in a multitude of ways. Hence, unlike other meats, you can eat fish just about every day and never get bored.

Beef

Although beef is generally considered to be high in saturated fat, it can be a relatively low-fat protein source—provided you choose the right types of meat. Certainly, porterhouse and chuck steaks are very fatty. Any meat on the bone or with a lot of marbling will fall into this category. But several cuts are actually quite lean. Sirloin, flank, and round steaks contain only moderate amounts of fat. Even better are game meats such as buffalo or venison which, because of their increased activity levels, tend to carry very low levels of adipose tissue. Regardless, make sure to trim all visible fat from the meats before cooking.

Eggs

One of the best sources of lean protein can be found in eggs. Due to a favorable profile of essential amino acids, eggs have the highest biological value (a popular measure of protein quality) of any whole-protein source. Egg protein is often the standard by which all other proteins are judged. Egg whites are the way to go, here. The whites are virtually pure protein; all the saturated fat is found in the yolk.

Milk

Milk is on par with eggs in terms of protein quality. There are two types of milk protein: casein and whey. Both types provide unique benefits and, because they digest at different speeds, are complementary when consumed in conjunction with each other. However, many people are lactose-intolerant (they lack the enzyme responsible for breaking down milk sugars) and therefore are unable to properly digest milk-based products. This can cause abdominal bloating and stomach cramps. What's more, since milk contains a fair amount of simple sugars, it can negatively impact insulin levels. Hence, milk proteins are best consumed in powdered form. In this way, they can be added to water, juice, or whole foods for a power-packed meal.

Soy

Last but not least, there is soy—a vegetable-based protein source. Although not as high quality as some other proteins, soy does contain a fairly good mix of essential amino acids (although it is a little low in methionine). Given that it isn't animal based, soy is the hands-down favorite protein of vegans and strict vegetarians.

Soy has also been touted as having health-promoting benefits. For one, it seems to promote positive effects on cardiovascular function. Studies have shown that regular soy consumption tends to lower LDL cholesterol, a primary risk factor in cardiovascular disease. This is attributed to its content of phytoestrogens—naturally occurring plant compounds that have weak estrogenic properties. Based on current evidence, soy does appear to be a heart-healthy product.

Less clear is the claim that soy is an anticarcinogen. On the one hand, several studies do show that soy helps to reduce the risk of various forms of cancer. Other studies, however, suggest that soy might actually promote tumor growth. Because of the phytoestrogens, breast tumors have actually increased in size when soy is given to women with breast cancer. It's not clear what to make of the conflicting aspects of the research, but the fact that there's even the potential for increasing cancer risk is cause for alarm.

Given the discrepancies in research, it is prudent to take a moderate approach to soy intake: Include soy as part of your diet, but refrain from consuming it on a daily basis. Until further studies clarify the facts, it's best to be cautious. While soy shows a great deal of promise as a healthful food, there are still more questions that need to be answered.

RECOMMENDED INTAKE

Protein should account for approximately 30 percent of total calories, equating to about one gram of protein per pound of body weight. Hence, a woman weighing 120 pounds needs to consume a minimum of 120 grams of protein per day. Any less and you risk falling into a negative nitrogen balance. Disregard the United States Department of Agriculture's recommended daily allowance (RDA) for protein (an absurdly low $\frac{4}{10}$ of a gram per pound of body weight). The RDA is based on the needs of sedentary people and doesn't take into account the increased protein demands of active individuals.

Make sure that your choice of proteins comes from lean sources. Skinless poultry breast, lean red meats, seafood, and egg whites are excellent choices. For convenience, there is a wide variety of protein powders available at health-food stores and other outlets.

Putting It All Together

Table 10.2 summarizes the nutritional protocols that will help you look great at any age. Use these protocols as a guideline and adapt them to your individual needs. As previously stated, every woman is unique. Hence, there is no single *best* nutritional program. Experiment with different nutrient ratios and see how it affects your body. Over time, you'll find out what works best for you.

Table 10.2

SUMMARY OF NUTRITIONAL PROTOCOLS		
Nutrient	**Recommended Percentage of Total Calories**	**Specific Recommendations**
Carbohydrates	40 to 50%	• Eat low-glycemic carbs. • Take in a high amount of fiber.
Protein	30 to 40%	• Eat lean, high-quality protein sources.
Fat	15 to 20%	• Eat mostly unsaturated, essential fatty acids.

CHAPTER 11

Tips to Stay Lean

The complexities of nutrition go beyond carbs, protein, and fat. While there's little doubt that the amount and proportion of these macronutrients are the dominant factors in weight management, other nutritional aspects also can have a significant impact on your physique. The following eight strategies and sample meal plans will help to elevate your metabolism and maximize your body's fat-burning ability. By integrating these principles into your nutritional approach, it's possible to achieve a leaner physique without altering caloric intake. This is especially pertinent when it comes to shedding those last few pounds that always seem so hard to get rid of.

EAT SMALL, FREQUENT MEALS

In today's fast-paced world, most women give little thought to the timing of their meals. All too often, breakfast consists of only a cup of coffee. Succeeding meals are eaten whenever there is a free moment, usually culminating in a large feast at dinner and possibly a midnight snack.

Unfortunately, this type of nutritional regimen has a deleterious effect on your body composition. When you deprive your body of food for more than a few hours, it senses that it won't have adequate fuel to carry out daily activities and shifts into a "starvation mode" as a means of conserving energy. Consequently, your metabolic rate slows down, preventing additional burning of calories. In addition, blood-sugar levels get out of whack. There is a tendency toward hypoglycemia, which causes hunger pangs and food cravings. Ultimately, this can promote binge eating and thereby pack on unwanted pounds.

By regimenting your eating patterns and consuming small, frequent meals, your body is able to operate at peak efficiency. Nutrients are better absorbed into your system, allowing them to be efficiently utilized for important biological functions. Your metabolism revs up which, in turn, helps to accelerate fat burning. Moreover, blood sugar remains stable, making you less likely to binge out on a big meal late in the day.

There is also an expenditure of energy in the digestion process, called dietary-induced thermogenesis. Every time you eat, your body burns off approximately 10 percent of the calories consumed, keeping your metabolism elevated for up to several hours after consumption. By constantly taking in food, you increase dietary-induced thermogenesis and thus maintain a raised metabolic rate throughout the day.

Ideally, you should space out your meals evenly, eating five or six times a day at regular intervals. While this might seem like a time-consuming chore, it actually can be accomplished without a great deal of effort. For instance, you can prepare several meals in advance, store them in Tupperware, and reheat them in a microwave on an as-needed basis. As an alternative, you can supplement your basic meals with powdered meal-replacements or sports bars. These "engineered foods" provide the ultimate in convenience: They are nutritionally balanced, easily transportable, and can be prepared in a matter of minutes.

DECREASE STARCHY CARBS AT NIGHT

For most women, starchy carbs make up a substantial portion of their evening meals. Pasta, rice, potatoes . . . these are nightly staples in the standard American diet. Steak and fries, spaghetti and meatballs—what would dinner be without them?

The trouble with starchy carbs is that they are readily transformed to fat when eaten before bedtime. The reason for this is simple: the primary function of carbohydrates is to supply short-term energy for your daily activities. If carbs are not used immediately for fuel, they have two possible fates: They either are stored as glycogen in your liver and muscles or are converted into fatty acids and stored in adipose tissue as body fat. Since activity levels usually are lowest during the evening hours, there is a diminished use of carbs for fuel and therefore an increased potential for body-fat storage.

In general, the best time to consume carbs is early in the day, when your activity levels are at their peak. This will allow your body to utilize a maximal amount of carbs for energy and minimize the potential for fat deposition. Breakfast, in particular, is an excellent time to load up on complex carbs. A large bowl of rolled oats or bran cereal will set the stage for fueling your daily activities and keep you physically and mentally fit throughout the day.

On the other hand, it is best to limit your dinner fare to fibrous, vegetable-based carbohydrate sources. Fiber-rich vegetables tend to be extremely low in total calories and, because of their bulk, are very filling. For supper, consider eating a meal consisting of lean poultry or fish combined with a large bowl of salad greens. Other vegetables such as broccoli, string beans, cauliflower, and zucchini also make fine nighttime carbohydrate choices and will reduce the potential for unwanted body-fat storage.

STAY HYDRATED

Believe it or not, most of your body is made up of water. Your muscles are roughly 75 percent water, your blood is more than 80 percent water, and your lungs are almost 90 percent water. Clearly, water is the most vital of all nutrients—without it, you would die in a matter of days.

Regrettably, some women cut back on their fluid intake, thinking that it will help to eliminate subcutaneous water retention. In some cases, they'll go so far as to refrain from drinking liquids altogether. This, however, is a big mistake! When fluids are restricted, your body senses a threat to its survival and tries to hold on to every last drop of water. The end result is an increase in water retention, leaving you puffy and bloated.

Worse, fluid restriction tends to make you fatter. Without an adequate supply of water, your kidney function becomes impaired, causing a systemic accumulation of metabolic waste. Your liver, in turn, has to work overtime to flush out these toxins from your body. This compromises your liver's ability to metabolize fat into usable energy—one of its primary responsibilities. As a result, less fat is metabolized, causing an increase in fat storage.

In order to avoid this fate, water should be readily consumed. Aim to drink three-quarters of an ounce of fluid per pound of body weight (based on your ideal body weight—what you aspire to weigh), spacing out intake throughout the day. Thus, if you weigh 120 pounds, you should consume approximately 90 ounces of water (a little under 3 quarts). Alcohol and caffeine-based beverages don't count toward this amount; they have a diuretic effect and actually cause you to dehydrate. Rather, your best bet is to drink plain old water, and a lot of it. Although tap water will suffice, natural spring water is a decidedly better choice. It is devoid of the pollutants that taint our reservoirs and therefore keeps your body free of contaminants. If possible, the water should be chilled or served on ice. Cold water is absorbed into the system more quickly than warm water, ensuring a continued state of hydration.

During exercise, fluid intake should be increased still further. As you work out, a large amount of water is lost through your sweat, breath, and urine. If these fluids aren't replenished, your exercise performance is bound to suffer. In fact, a mere 3 percent reduction in water can cause up to a 10 percent loss in muscular strength. When taken to the extreme, heatstroke or even circulatory collapse can occur. Clearly, exercise-induced dehydration must be avoided at all costs.

It is a mistake, however, to rely on thirst as an indicator as to when to drink. Intense exercise inhibits the thirst sensors in your throat and gut; by the time you become thirsty, your body already is severely dehydrated. Therefore, during exercise, drink early and drink often. Consume eight ounces of fluid immediately before your workout and then take small sips of water every five or ten minutes or so while training.

GO EASY ON THE SAUCE

The world floats on a sea of alcohol. Whether it's the two-martini lunch, the evening happy hour, or the after-dinner drink, alcohol is firmly ingrained in today's society. It is, without question, the most popular recreational drug in existence. In many circles, getting drunk is even a rite of passage—a rite that often continues throughout adulthood. With such widespread social acceptance, it's no wonder that approximately half of all Americans drink on a regular basis and more than 5 percent are heavy drinkers.

However, for any woman who aspires to maximize her body's potential, excessive alcohol consumption is a definite taboo. Make no mistake: Alcohol will make you fat. It is calorically dense, containing over 7 calories per gram (as opposed to carbs and protein, which have 4). And this doesn't include the addition of mixers, which can significantly increase the calorie count. Take a look at the caloric content in some popular alcoholic beverages: a margarita has 600 calories, a martini 250, and a beer 150—pretty heavy stuff! What's more, these drinks are virtually devoid of any nutritional value. They are "empty calories" that do nothing but pack on unwanted pounds. Considering these facts, there is no doubt that even moderate drinking can have a decidedly negative impact on your figure.

Moreover, it is difficult for the body to break down alcohol. The liver must use a tremendous amount of coenzymes (such as NAD and FAD) in order to assimilate the toxins from alcohol. Consequently, there are fewer coenzymes available to carry out vital metabolic functions, including the breakdown of fat for energy. The end result: increased fat storage. This process can begin after just a single night of heavy drinking.

With chronic abuse, the consequences of alcohol can be disastrous—often irreparable. Alcohol is a poison. It infiltrates your internal organs and has a toxic effect on everything that it comes into contact with. Your liver and spleen, in particular, become severely impaired and lose their ability to carry out vital functions. Forget about losing body fat; your entire metabolic system becomes dysfunctional. And don't think your muscles are immune from the carnage. Sustained bouts of heavy drinking ultimately cause myopathy— a degeneration of muscle tissue that obliterates your hard-earned gains.

The best advice on alcohol is to limit consumption to no more than one drink a day. Get used to the idea that you don't need alcohol to have a good time. If you're out at a party or dance club, order a club soda with a twist of lemon or lime. Once you have adjusted to being a teetotaler, you'll soon appreciate the associated benefits. When others are in a drunken stupor, you'll be in full control of your faculties. You'll wake up hangover-free, never having to regret what you did the night before. And, of course, you'll keep your body operating at peak efficiency, maintaining optimal shape year round.

HOLD THE SALT

Salt is the most widely used of all spices. It is added to almost every food imaginable: from soup to nuts and everything in between.

The craving for salt is physiologic. You see, there are distinct taste buds that reside on the tip and upper front portion of the tongue, that are specifically receptive to salty foods.

Salt is composed of sodium (as well as chloride), a basic mineral that's abundant in nature. Because it carries an electrical charge, sodium is considered an *electrolyte*. In conjunction with potassium, it is responsible for regulating the body's fluid balance; potassium maintains the fluid balance intracellularly (within the cells), while sodium maintains the balance of fluids extracellularly (outside of the cells). Hence, sodium is essential for bodily function; a lack of it leads to hyponatremia, a condition that ultimately causes death.

Although it is an essential nutrient, only minute quantities of sodium are required through dietary means. In fact, a mere 500 milligrams is all that's needed to maintain normal biologic function—an amount that equates to about a quarter teaspoon of salt. Yet the average American consumes more than ten times this quantity! When too much sodium is ingested, fluid is drawn out of the cells and into the body's free spaces, causing the malady known as water retention. Your feet and hands swell, your face becomes puffy, and water accumulates beneath your skin: not an enviable condition for someone trying to maintain a lean, toned physique. The fact is, sodium occurs naturally in most foods, and you'll get all you need just by eating a sensible diet.

The best way to avoid an overconsumption of sodium is by eating fresh, unprocessed foods. Stay away from all prepackaged and canned goods. They tend to be the worst offenders. Many condiments and sauces also are loaded with sodium. Ketchup, salad dressings, and soy sauce all contain whopping amounts. And in order to avoid any hidden sources, get used to reading food labels. The sodium content is plainly listed for all to see.

In addition, refrain from adding salt to your meals. If you want to spice up your foods, there are dozens of delicious seasonings that can enhance flavor without any side effects. Paprika, cinnamon, basil, oregano, garlic—the list goes on. Experiment with different combinations and see what you find palatable. By using a little ingenuity, you can create tasty dishes that are virtually sodium-free.

JUMP-START WITH JAVA

Caffeine has gotten a bad rap. For years, health-care practitioners have denounced it as a health hazard. They've cautioned against its use, citing studies that link it to everything from heart disease to cancer. However, the bulk of these studies were flawed in their design. Some used enormous quantities of caffeine—far beyond what the normal individual consumes. Others employed insufficient sample sizes or had errors in statistical analysis. The truth is, when all the available information is examined, there's really no evidence that modest caffeine consumption causes any detriments to overall health and well-being. In fact, a few studies actually found a negative correlation between caffeine and certain forms of cancer!

Does this mean that you should load up on caffeinated beverages? Absolutely not! Caffeine is a stimulant. At high doses, it can cause a host of unwanted side effects such as hypertension, nervousness, insomnia, and gastrointestinal distress. Guzzling mass quantities of coffee and cola will only serve to make you wired and irritable—not lean and defined.

However, when used in moderation, caffeine can be a safe and effective means of expediting a loss of body fat. By stimulating catecholamines (adrenaline and noradrenaline), caffeine facilitates the release of free fatty acids from fat cells, allowing fat to be utilized for short-term energy. Studies have shown up to a 4 percent increase in resting metabolic rate from judicious caffeine supplementation, with effects lasting up to several hours after ingestion.

You don't need to take a lot of caffeine to derive positive benefits. A daily dose of 200 to 300 milligrams is all that's required to rev up your metabolic rate. Two cups of brewed coffee first thing in the morning will satisfy this requirement quite nicely. Better yet, consume the coffee immediately before your workout. In addition to its fat-burning effects, caffeine helps to delay fatigue and improve exercise intensity. Your performance will be enhanced, spurring you on to greater gains.

But remember to avoid going overboard with caffeine consumption. Excessive intake has no additional benefits and can actually impede results. When consumed in abundance, caffeine acts as a *vasoconstrictor,* narrowing arteries and restricting blood flow. As you may recall, a reduced circulatory capacity inhibits the breakdown of stored body fat. Ultimately, this counteracts the thermogenic effects of caffeine, nullifying its fat-burning benefits.

For best results, black coffee or espresso is recommended; adding cream or sugar will easily offset the caffeine-induced increase in metabolic rate. If black coffee is simply too bitter for your taste buds, then try using skim milk and artificial sweeteners as flavor enhancers.

An even better alternative to coffee is green tea. In addition to having caffeine, green tea contains special compounds called catechin polyphenols that increase the thermogenic effect of caffeine. Catechins inhibit an enzyme (called catechol-O-methyl transferase) that degrades noradrenaline, a potent hormone that promotes the mobilization of body fat. In combination, caffeine and catechins act synergistically, enhancing resting energy expenditure beyond that of caffeine alone. Considering that it also is replete with vitamins and antioxidants (the benefits of which are discussed in the next section), green tea is a terrific beverage for keeping your body healthy and lean.

HAVE AN ANTIOXIDANT COCKTAIL

Much has been made about vitamin and mineral supplementation. For many generations, these so-called micronutrients were touted as wonder supplements, heralded for curing everything from the common cold to night blindness. While we now know these claims to be greatly exaggerated, this doesn't diminish the fact that micronutrients are imperative for maintaining a fit, healthy body.

Vitamins and minerals serve many important biological functions. They facilitate energy transfer, prevent disease, and act as coenzymes to assist in many chemical reactions. A deficiency in any of these micronutrients can lead to severe illness. While you likely will get the Recommended Dietary Allowance of all micronutrients by following my dietary recommendations, there might be cases (depending on food choices and total caloric intake) where a deficiency could arise. Thus, it is a good idea to take a multivitamin/mineral complex. This acts as an insurance policy, guaranteeing that all your needs are met.

There is a special class of micronutrients called antioxidants that are required in much larger amounts than other vitamins and minerals. Antioxidants are the body's scavengers. They help to defend the body against damage caused by free radicals—unstable molecules that can injure healthy cells and tissues. Millions of these dangerous villains are produced each day during the normal course of respiration. The main culprit: oxygen. Every time you breathe, oxygen uptake causes free radical production. Environmental factors such as pollutants, smoke, and certain chemicals also contribute to their formation. If left unchecked, free radicals can wreak havoc on your physique and cause a multitude of ailments including arthritis, cardiovascular disease, dementia, and cancer.

For the active woman, antioxidants are of particular importance. Due to increased oxygen consumption, free radical production skyrockets during exercise. This results in an inflammation of muscle tissue, impairing muscular function and slowing recovery. The capacity for muscular repair is reduced, heightening the likelihood of overtraining.

Fortunately, like heroic warriors, antioxidants engulf free radicals, rendering them harmless. Not only does this improve your overall health and well-being, but it also improves your exercise capacity. There is a reduction in postexercise muscle inflammation (with an associated decrease in delayed-onset muscle soreness), helping to repair bodily tissues and speed recovery.

While there are dozens of known antioxidants, four of them are absolutely indispensable: vitamin C, vitamin E, coenzyme Q10, and alpha-lipoic acid. These antioxidants work synergistically with one another; their combined effect is greater than the sum of their individual actions. Other antioxidants that are beneficial include selenium, lycopene, isoflavones, and polyphenols (although they don't have the synergistic capabilities of the "big four").

It is virtually impossible, however, to consume adequate quantities of antioxidants from food sources. For example, you'd have to drink eleven glasses of orange juice in order to get the recommended amount of vitamin C. Hence, supplementation is an absolute necessity. Table 11.1 lists the major antioxidants with corresponding dosages.

As a rule, it is best to consume supplements in conjunction with a meal. The absorption of micronutrients is improved when they are consumed with food. This also improves gastrointestinal tolerance of the supplement.

Table 11.1

ANTIOXIDANT	DOSAGE
VITAMIN C	800 mg
VITAMIN E	600 IU
COENZYME Q10	50 mg
ALPHA-LIPOIC ACID	100 mg
POLYPHENOLS	50 mg
SOY ISOFLAVONES	50 mg
LYCOPENE	10 mg
SELENIUM	200 mcg

CHEAT A LITTLE

Throughout the ages, food has always been a source of great temptation. Dating all the way back to Adam and Eve, there was the forbidden fruit; that luscious apple was simply too much to resist. Today, with food so plentiful, the temptations are literally endless. Let's face it, a great deal of willpower is required to pass up a slice of birthday cake or forgo a bucket of chicken wings. For some, the thought of never again eating these types of foods is too much to bear. After several months of deprivation, they break down and go on an eating binge, scarfing down everything in sight.

To help keep your sanity, it is acceptable—even beneficial—to have a "cheat" day. On your cheat day, you can eat basically anything you want including sugar- and/or fat-laden foods. Within reason, there are no restrictions. Go ahead and order a pizza. Frequent your favorite fast-food restaurant. Have a candy bar. Whatever you heart desires, feel free to indulge. You don't need to feel guilty about cheating; consider it a reward for sticking to your diet.

Try not to go too far overboard, though. While a little overindulgence won't have any effect on your physique, consuming mass quantities of food very well could (and it also can make you pretty sick!). Accordingly, don't allow the total calories on your cheat day to exceed more than 150 percent of your estimated daily intake. For instance, if you normally eat 1,600 calories, don't go past 2,400 calories. This will give you plenty of leeway to satisfy your food cravings while keeping caloric intake within a reasonable range.

Finally, make sure to limit cheating to no more than one day per week. Try to pick a specific cheat day and stay with it. Regimentation is an important part of maintaining a healthy lifestyle and when cheating becomes a habit, regimentation goes by the wayside. Stick with the program and make your cheat day a special treat.

CHAPTER 12

Sample Meal Plans

In this chapter, you will find one-week sample menus based on the High-Energy Fitness™ nutritional protocols outlined in this book. There are six days of well-organized menus, with strict control of calories and proper nutrient partitioning. The daily meals are based on a 1,500-calorie diet. Based on your individual needs and goals, you might need to adjust the caloric intake slightly. Just make sure to keep the basic principles intact, maintaining the approximate macronutrient profile outlined in Table 10.2 on page 133. Day 7 is your cheat day: your reward for staying regimented throughout the week. On your cheat day, eat whatever you want and enjoy!

Monday

MEAL ONE
- 6 egg whites, scrambled
- 1 medium whole-wheat bagel
- 1 cup green tea

MEAL TWO
- 1 ounce mixed nuts

MEAL THREE
- Tuna salad (6 ounces tuna in water, 1 cup romaine lettuce, 1 tomato, 1 tablespoon olive oil)
- 1 medium sweet potato
- 1 cup green tea

MEAL FOUR
- 1 medium pear

MEAL FIVE
- 6 ounces grilled chicken breast
- 12 ounces steamed cauliflower

1,469 calories
Carbohydrate: 149 grams (40 percent)
Protein: 144 grams (39 percent)
Fat: 34 grams (21 percent)

Tuesday

MEAL ONE
- 1 cup Special K cereal served with 4 ounces skim milk and 1 ounce seedless raisins
- 1 cup orange juice
- 1 cup green tea

MEAL TWO
- 1 medium apple

MEAL THREE
- Turkey sandwich (6 ounces turkey breast, 2 slices whole-wheat bread, mustard)
- Large salad (1 cup romaine lettuce, 1 tomato, 1 tablespoon olive oil)
- 1 cup green tea

MEAL FOUR
- Meal replacement shake (consisting of 37 grams of protein and 22 grams of carbohydrate, such as MET-Rx, Myoplex, Rx Fuel, etc.)

MEAL FIVE
- 4 ounces broiled salmon
- 12 ounces steamed broccoli

1,441 calories
Carbohydrate: 170 grams (46 percent)
Protein: 125 grams (34 percent)
Fat: 34 grams (20 percent)

Wednesday

MEAL ONE
- 8 ounces instant Cream of Wheat
- 1 tablespoon flaxseed oil
- 1 scoop whey protein powder (mixed in water or into the oatmeal)
- 1 cup green tea

MEAL TWO
- 1 medium banana

MEAL THREE
- 1 cup (dry weight) brown rice
- 4 ounces baked flounder
- Large salad (1 cup romaine lettuce, 1 tomato, 1 serving fat-free dressing of choice)
- 1 cup green tea

MEAL FOUR
- 8 ounces plain, nonfat yogurt

MEAL FIVE
- 6 ounces broiled sirloin steak
- 12 ounces steamed asparagus

1,505 calories
Carbohydrate: 159 grams (42 percent)
Protein: 131 grams (34 percent)
Fat: 41 grams (24 percent)

Thursday

MEAL ONE
- 1 cup instant oatmeal
- 1 scoop whey protein powder
- 8-ounce glass fresh cranberry juice
- 1 cup green tea

MEAL TWO
- 1.5 ounces roasted almonds

MEAL THREE
- 6-ounce turkey burger on rye
- Large salad (1 cup romaine lettuce, 1 tomato,
  1 serving fat-free dressing of choice)
- 1 cup green tea

MEAL FOUR
- 2 cups fresh strawberries

MEAL FIVE
- 6 ounces grilled shrimp
- 12 ounces steamed spinach

1,455 calories
Carbohydrate: 160 grams (41 percent)
Protein: 141 grams (37 percent)
Fat: 37 grams (22 percent)

Friday

MEAL ONE
- 1 medium whole-wheat bagel
- 6 ounces cottage cheese
- 1 cup green tea

MEAL TWO
• 1 medium orange

MEAL THREE
• 6 ounces chili con carne
• Large salad (1 cup romaine lettuce, 1 tomato, 1 tablespoon olive oil)
• 1 cup green tea

MEAL FOUR
• Meal replacement shake (consisting of 37 grams of protein and 22 grams of carbohydrate)

MEAL FIVE
• 6 ounces broiled tofu
• 12 ounces steamed green beans

1,410 calories
Carbohydrate: 146 grams (40 percent)
Protein: 121 grams (33 percent)
Fat: 44 grams (27 percent)

Saturday

MEAL ONE
• Power pancakes (1 cup complete whole-wheat pancake mix, 1 scoop whey protein powder, and 1 cup water)

MEAL TWO
• Strawberry protein smoothie (2 cups strawberries, 2 scoops soy protein powder, and 1 cup water)

MEAL THREE
• Black bean salad (1 cup black beans, 1 cup romaine lettuce, 1 tomato, and 1 tablespoon olive oil)

MEAL FOUR
• 2 medium peaches

MEAL FIVE
- 6 ounces broiled trout
- 12 ounces grilled zucchini

1,436 calories

Carbohydrate: 160 grams (44 percent)

Protein: 129 grams (35 percent)

Fat: 35 grams (21 percent)

High-Fiber Foods

FOOD	AMOUNT	FIBER CONTENT (G)
APPLE	Medium	3
ALL-BRAN CEREAL	1 ounce	10
BARLEY	1 cup	6
BLACKBERRIES	1 cup	8
BLACK BEANS	1 cup	19
BREAD (WHOLE WHEAT)	2 slices	6
BROCCOLI	1 cup	8
CHICKPEAS	1 cup	12

FOOD	AMOUNT	FIBER CONTENT (G)
CORN	Medium	5
GREEN PEAS	1 cup	18
LENTILS	1 cup	15
OATMEAL	½ cup	4
PEAR	Medium	4
RASPBERRIES	1 cup	9
RICE (BROWN)	½ cup	5
SPINACH	1 cup	7
YAMS	Medium	7

Glossary of Fitness Terms

Adipocyte. Fat cell.

Aerobic Exericse. Any activity that allows your body to consistently replenish oxygen to your working muscles. It is performed at a low to moderate intensity and is endurance oriented by nature. Both fat and glycogen are burned for fuel.

Alpha-2 Receptor. "Entrance" that allows fat to enter an adipocyte.

Anaerobic Exercise. Any activity that utilizes oxygen at a faster rate than your body can replenish it in the working muscles. By nature, this type of exercise is intense and short in duration. Glycogen is the primary source of fuel.

Barbell. A long bar, usually measuring about six feet in length, that can accommodate weighted plates on each end. The Olympic barbell is the industry standard and weighs forty-five pounds.

Bench. An apparatus designed for performing exercises in a seated or lying fashion. Many benches are adjustable so that exercises can be performed at a wide array of different angles.

Beta Receptor. "Exit" that allows fat to escape an adipocyte.

Body Sculpting. The art of shaping your muscles to optimal proportions.

Cardio. Short for cardiovascular (aerobic) exercise.

Circuit Training. A series of exercise machines set up in sequence. The exercises are performed one after the other, each stressing a different muscle group.

Collar. A clamp that secures weighted plates on a barbell or dumbbell.

Compound Movement. An exercise that involves two or more joints in the performance of the movement. Examples include squats, bench presses, and chins.

Contraction. The act of shortening a muscle.

Cross Training. Using two or more different exercises in a routine. Generally used in the context of aerobic activities.

Definition. The absence of fat in the presence of well-developed muscle.

Dumbbell. A shortened version of a barbell, usually measuring about twelve inches in length, that allows an exercise to be performed one arm at a time.

Estrogen. Primary female hormone. Linked to increased fat storage.

Exercise. An individual movement that is intended to tax muscular function.

Failure. The point in an exercise where you cannot physically perform another rep.

Flexibility. A litheness of the joints, muscle, and connective tissue that dictates range of motion.

Form. The technique utilized in performing the biomechanics of an exercise.

Free Weights. Barbells and dumbbells. This is opposed to exercise machines.

Hypertrophy. An increase in muscle mass.

Intensity. The amount of effort involved in a set.

Isolation Movement. An exercise that involves only one joint in the performance of the movement. Examples include cable crossovers, biceps curls, and leg extensions.

Nautilus. A brand of exercise equipment found in many health clubs. The term has become synonymous with any exercise machine.

Plates. Flat, round weights that can be placed at the end of a barbell or dumbbell.

Progesterone. Primary female hormone. Linked to increased appetite.

Pump. The pooling of blood in a muscle due to intense anaerobic exercise.

Repetition (Rep). One complete movement of an exercise.

Resistance. The amount of weight used in an exercise.

Rest Interval. The amount of time taken in between sets.

Routine. The configuration of exercises, sets, and reps that one utilizes in a training session.

Set. A series of repetitions performed in succession.

Symmetry. The way in which muscle groups complement one another, creating a proportional physique.

Testosterone. A hormone that is responsible for promoting muscle mass.

Thermogenesis. Increased body heat. Accelerates fat burning.

Index

Index

About the Author

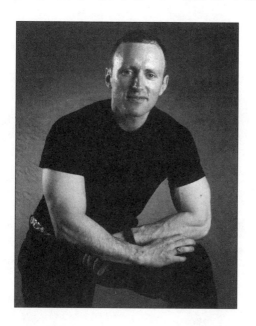

Brad Schoenfeld is widely regarded as one of America's leading health and fitness experts. He is the author of the best-selling fitness books *Look Great Naked, Look Great Sleeveless,* and *Sculpting Her Body Perfect*. He has been published or featured in virtually every major magazine (including *Cosmopolitan, Self, Marie Claire, Fitness,* and *Shape*) and has appeared on hundreds of television shows and radio programs across the United States. Certified as a strength and conditioning specialist (by the National Strength and Conditioning Association) and as a personal trainer (by both the American Council on Exercise and the Aerobics and Fitness Association of America), Schoenfeld was awarded the distinction of being classified as a Master Trainer by the International Association of Fitness Professionals. He is also the producer of three videos that feature his Look Great program (*Look Great Naked Abs, Look Great Naked Butt,* and *Look Great Naked Thighs*) and runs the Web site www.lookgreatnaked.com. A frequent lecturer on both the professional and consumer level, Schoenfeld is owner/operator of the exclusive Personal Training Center for Women in Scarsdale, New York. He lives in Croton-on-Hudson, New York.

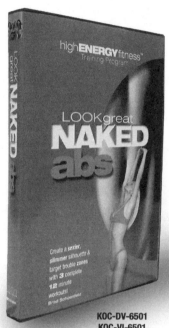
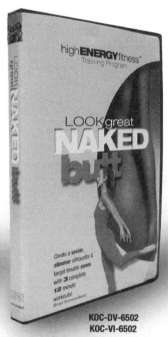
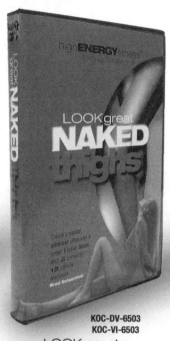
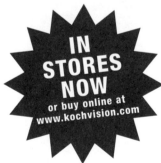

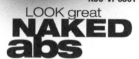